LOCAL WOMEN, GLOBAL SCIENCE

Local Women, Global Science

Fighting AIDS in Kenya

Karen M. Booth

INDIANA UNIVERSITY PRESS

Bloomington and Indianapolis

Publication of this book is made possible in part with the assistance of a Challenge Grant from
the National Endowment for the Humanities, a federal agency that supports research, education,
and public programming in the humanities.

This book is a publication of

Indiana University Press

601 North Morton Street
Bloomington, Indiana 47404-3797 USA

http://iupress.indiana.edu

Telephone orders	800-842-6796
Fax orders	812-855-7931
Orders by e-mail	iuporder@indiana.edu

© 2004 by Karen M. Booth

The paper used in this publication meets the minimum requirements of American National
Standard for Information Sciences—Permanence of Paper for Printed Library Materials,
ANSI Z39.48-1984.

Manufactured in the United States of America

Library of Congress Cataloging-in-Publication Data

Booth, Karen M., date
Local women, global science : fighting AIDS in Kenya / Karen M. Booth.
p.   cm.
Includes bibliographical references and index.
ISBN 0-253-34181-7 (cloth : alk. paper) — ISBN 0-253-21640-0 (paper : alk. paper)
1. AIDS (Disease)—Kenya. 2. AIDS (Disease) in women—Kenya. 3. AIDS
(Disease)—Government policy.

[DNLM: 1. HIV Infections—prevention & control—Kenya. 2. HIV
Infections—ethnology—Kenya. 3. Health Policy—Kenya. 4. Sex
Behavior—ethnology—Kenya. 5. Women's Health—Kenya. 6. Women's Rights—Kenya.
WC 503.6 B725L 2004] I. Title.
RA643.86.K4B667 2004
362.1′969792′0096762—dc21
2003011796

1 2 3 4 5   09 08 07 06 05 04

Contents

Acknowledgments

Over the course of the noncontiguous times and spaces in which I designed this study, did the fieldwork, and analyzed, wrote, and rewrote this story, I have depended on and learned from many generous and amazing people, each of whom has been my teacher in some way. I began the process in Madison, Wisconsin, where Alberto Palloni and Gay Seidman encouraged, supported, and defended my work while mentoring me in so many ways. Alberto let me cry over the phone and then helped me reconnect with my passion and goals while I was in Geneva waiting for the Kenyan government to give me permission to do my research. The wisdom, patience, and humor with which he responded to my fumbling analyses and theorizing grounded me. Gay's tireless efforts to help me write through and beyond my confusion enabled me to finish the dissertation then. Her not-always-gentle but endlessly constructive and loving guidance has become a part of my current practice as a scholar and teacher. Aili Tripp, Joanne Csete, and the late Elaine Marks each helped me develop specific skills that have been crucial in this process. All three also became friends and examples of scholars whose research and teaching are or were consistently informed by their feminist politics. Magdalena Hauner helped me fall in love with Kiswahili.

Through the Institute of Global Studies at the University of Wisconsin, the John D. and Catherine T. MacArthur Foundation funded my year of proposal writing and one year of writing. During this time, the foundation supported the creation of the "Gender Network," which brought together MacArthur scholars from the University of Wisconsin, the University of Minnesota, and Stanford University. This group viii

created a community that sustained me. The foundation and the institute also gave me a wonderful job with an office and computer that made finishing my dissertation possible. I thank David Trubeck and Jim Riker at the institute for their support.

As part of their program on African health and agriculture, funded by the Ford Foundation, the Social Science Research Council (SSRC) gave me a very generous dissertation grant. With this grant I was able to get short-term training at the Johns Hopkins School of Hygiene and Public Health and two and one-half years of field work in Kenya and Geneva. This grant program supported crucial research on key issues in a region of the world perceived by the U.S. government then and now to be without value. I am grateful to the SSRC for its integrity, commitment, and foresight. At Johns Hopkins, Barbara de Zalduondo and Purnima Mane helped me make the sometimes large leap between anthropological and medical ways of telling stories.

I do not know how many of my friends, supporters, and contributors in Nairobi will read this book. I hope that in some small way my story will call more attention to the integrity, intelligence, dedication, and generosity of the many nurses who were my teachers at the University of Nairobi, the Nairobi Special Treatment Clinic (Casino), and the peripheral health center that I have here called "Bestlands." They are the center of my story. They were the center and the highlight of my fieldwork. I could not begin to catalog all of the things about health, sexuality, gender, and community that I learned from them. Their laughter, even when it was directed at me, was wonderful. Their perceptions and analyses were marvelous and so generously given. They remain anonymous here only because I do not wish in any way to cause embarrassment or trouble for any individual. I do believe, however, that if my book is read in the way that I intended (which is never a guarantee), the integrity, honesty, and ability of these women to provide good care in the face of severe crisis will be clear. I also thank the many patients who had no idea who this strange white woman was or why I was listening to them but who went ahead and told their stories anyway.

Thanks largely to Elizabeth Ngugi's generosity and interest in my work, I was welcomed by the Department of Community Health at the University of Nairobi and by the Nairobi HIV/STD Project. I could not have done this project if they had not admitted me and if Dr. Ngugi had not paved my way into the clinics. Although in this book I am critical of many aspects of this project, I am impressed by Dr. Ngugi's unusual commitment to stopping the spread of HIV among some of the world's most marginalized women. She and her staff listened to women who had never before been considered an important constituency deserving attention, counseling, and good health care. Her remarkable work among Nairobi's sex workers and adolescents has deservedly become a model of peer-based HIV interventions in many parts of the world. Her staff, especially Ruth Ketyenya, Anastasia Ndiritu, and Catherine Ngugi, showed me the way around and answered all of my no-doubt-annoying questions with patience and wisdom. Gloria Eldridge, a member of the team from the Canadian International Development Agency, befriended me and helped me see that the project, and HIV itself, were more complicated than I believed. Gloria was absolutely crucial to my ability to keep hoping and laughing in the midst of Nairobi's terrible crises.

Roselyn Ochieng and Paul Saoke gave me a home and a family. When I arrived, Paul tracked me down and insisted that I move from the grubby hotel in which I had expected to live out my fieldwork days to his home and to the lives of 6-year-old Beryl Ochieng, newborn Alex Saoke, and their parents, cousins, aunts, and uncles. Every day I would get back to this home as soon as I could. There I would find laughter; play; intellectual conversation; lessons in cooking, language, politics, laundry, and music; poetry readings; updates on the latest demonstrations and strikes; and new friends. This home and this family enriched my time in Nairobi, my understanding of Kenyan politics, this book, and my life. I am grateful to Leslie McCall for introducing me to Paul.

I gave the World Health Organization's Global Programme on AIDS (GPA) a bit of a hard time. Catherine Dasen, a director of public information there, told me that I could not come as an "intern" when I asked to be given permission to do some research. When I showed up at her door anyway, she was confused but gracious and very helpful. I am grateful to her for giving me many important documents and for suggesting which members of the staff I might be most interested in interviewing. I was underfoot for months at the World Health Organization library, but Zoila Watters was so patient and so knowledgeable that I was able to get everything I needed and finish my work there surprisingly quickly. She also made poring over the technical language of United Nations documents pleasant, which was quite a feat.

One of my most important teachers was Priscilla Alexander, then the GPA's consultant on sex workers and both before and since that time a leader in the struggles to organize sex workers in the United States and worldwide. By telling me about her experiences, introducing me to key staff members, and letting me hang out in her office, at lunch in the cafeteria, and at various meetings, Priscilla allowed me to go behind the official, "technical," face of the GPA. She became my friend, sharing with me her passion for sex workers' rights, her commitment to getting feminists to see prostitutes as feminist activists and to become their allies rather than their enemies, and her home. Priscilla defines the word "activist"; she has given her life to the struggle for sexual liberation. She is an inspiration and a touchstone for me, modeling a standard to which I aspire and against which I measure my own commitment to making change. I also want to thank Kathleen Cravero, not only because she generously gave me both time and wonderful insights but also because of her determination to give the Global Programme on AIDS a feminist conscience.

The University of North Carolina at Chapel Hill helped to fund me as I wrote the book. I thank the University Research Council and the Purdue fellowship granted through the Institute for Arts and Humanities for this assistance. My colleagues and friends in Women's Studies, especially Barbara Harris, Jane Burns, Karen Thompson, and Donna Redford, have been patient, supportive, and caring throughout this process.

I want to thank my family and friends, those who have seen me through the highs and lows of this long process and continued to love me nonetheless. My parents, Mary Lou and Newell Booth, gave me financial help when I really needed it. More important, they have encouraged me, particularly during my struggles to transform this apparently unwieldy story into a book. Few are lucky enough to have a mentor who is also a sister and a friend. Marilyn Booth has been a constant source of wisdom, empathy, and wonderful ideas. Her passion for research, her brilliant writing, and her feminist politics have inspired me. Her "big sister" strategies have kept me going. Marie Ferré has been a rock.

Rachel Schurman has seen it all. She has been my teacher since the day I arrived at graduate school and was told to "age-adjust this population." She has taught me much more than practical and face-saving statistics, however. She has shown me how privilege and oppression operate at the international level, how to think politically and sociologically, and how to judge whether a piece of knowledge is "good" based not simply on how it was produced but also on whether it contributes to the making of a more just world.

Many other friends have made this book, and the fact that I have survived it, possible. The MacArthur Gender Network introduced me to Elisabeth Friedman, Nilgün Uygun, Jennifer Pierce, and the late and so-much-missed Susan Geiger. These amazing women have given me constructive feedback, intellectual and emotional support, and a lot of good times. Barrie Thorne, Carole Joffe, Raka Ray, Sherryl Kleinman, and Rashmi Varma have urged me on, reading my work and reminding me by their brilliance and caring of the kind of feminist scholar and teacher I want to be. Sherryl Kleinman and Rashmi Varma have also allowed me to complain while keeping me moving and laughing. Marianne Cutler did some important research and offered useful insights as well as friendship. Mindy Oshrain was there for me when I could not be there for myself, when I wanted to quit, and when I could not see where I was going or why. Quite literally this book would not have happened without her guidance. I am so grateful for the wonderful ideas and the helpful feedback that I have gotten from Michael Goldman, Judith Farquhuar, Stephen Ellis, Mary Layoun, Jane Collins, Cynthia Ofstead, and several anonymous reviewers. Thad, Leila, and my writing comrades at the Regulator Café in Durham gave me a wonderful community and great coffee. My amazing editor at Indiana, Dee Mortensen, has made it all happen right on time. Kate Babbitt and Jane Lyle provided superb technical support.

Finally and especially I want to thank Elyse Crystall, who has been my favorite and toughest teacher as well as my home for eight years. I am grateful for her patience, her fabulous sense of humor, and the nudges she gave me just when I needed them. Her inspiration, advice, insight, political commitment, and love are woven into this book, which is so much better and richer as a result.

Note on Terminology

I use the terms HIV, HIV/AIDS, and AIDS somewhat idiosyncratically to refer to three conceptually distinct dimensions and collective and individual experiences of the crisis. HIV refers to the virus that damages an infected individual's immune system and renders her vulnerable to a myriad of diseases and ultimately to death. I use HIV/AIDS to describe the total disease experience of people who are infected with HIV and those who are ill from any of the diseases that result from HIV infection. Finally, I reserve the use of the term AIDS to refer to the social constructions or representations of the collective experience of HIV infection and related illnesses.

LOCAL WOMEN, GLOBAL SCIENCE

One

Global Medicine, Local Sex, and Crisis

During the last few months of my fieldwork in Kenya, I had two quite different conversations that offer a starting point for this story about the politics of HIV. One of these conversations took place in a public primary health care center located on the city's periphery. The other happened downtown, just adjacent to the bustling and wealthy tourist-oriented part of Nairobi, in what was at the time the country's only government-run freestanding clinic treating sexually transmitted infections.

When the first conversation began, I was sitting in Room 2 at Bestlands Health Center, which provides the neighborhood (or "estate," as they call them in Kenya) of the same name with basic curative and preventive health care services.[1] The sister-in-charge,[2] the two nurses responsible for treating and counseling patients with sexually transmitted diseases (STDs), and I had just finished listening to a woman who had gonorrhea. After the woman swallowed her pills and left, I asked for a translation of the conversation with the patient.[3] As Wamuuchi, one of the STD nurses, started to give me a summary in English, Sister Kiroro jumped in, sounding angry. Glaring out the window at the mixture of concrete, tin, and mud-and-newspaper homes that made up her center's catchment area, she said: "A husband can have a thousand girlfriends. There's nothing an African woman can do!"[4]

I had understood enough of the interchange between the nurses and the gonorrhea patient to know that the latter had returned with the same complaint for which she had been treated several months before. The woman's apparent reinfection suggested that her husband had

1

never come in to be treated for the gonorrhea that he presumably had and was repeatedly transmitting to his wife. Looking directly at me now, Sister Kiroro went on: "One of the [project's] *Wazungu* [Europeans] came the other day and advised us to 'tell women to sleep on the couch or at the neighbor's house' if the husbands refused to get treated or use a condom." At this, Wamuuchi and the other STD nurse, Alice, started to laugh and nod their heads in agreement. Sister Kiroro turned to them and laughed too. "Can you imagine? What would your neighbors say? How would you explain that to your children? They would think you are crazy!" She stopped laughing and turned back to me: "Here," she said with emphasis, "a woman if she tries to say no [to sexual intercourse], she can be beaten or even thrown out."[5]

The second conversation actually took place several months earlier. I was standing in what was referred to as the "female hallway" of Nairobi's clinic for STDs, popularly known as Casino.[6] I was talking to several nurses there following the "healthy talk" they occasionally gave to the women and children waiting to be examined. I asked the nurses who had delivered the twenty-minute lecture why so few of the patients had taken the *condomi* which the nurses passed around at the end of the talk. Janet, the nurse who had participated in the talk mainly by miming—to some barely repressed laughter from the audience—how the patients should wash "*huku chini kila siku*" (down there every day), replied: "They do not really use them; the ones who will use, they take. But the others . . . You know anyway the condom is for the man. He has to agree." I nodded. I had heard this many times. "But anyway," she went on, "they say that the condom does not even prevent . . . it was in the paper the other day that the condom is not effective. We tell them to use it but now we don't know anymore. Should we even tell them to use it?" Nancy, the nurse who had run the healthy talk, nodded her agreement.[7]

The comments that Sister Kiroro and Janet made while they tried to do their work at Bestlands and Casino suggested to me that as they struggled to cope with HIV/AIDS, these nurses confronted three important and as-yet-unresolved problems. First, they perceived "African"[8] men's (hetero)sexual appetite to be insatiable; the nurses' words and practices indicated that they believed that neither infection nor the risk of infection curbs men's sexual appetites. Second, the nurses viewed "African" women as powerless, victims of the heterosexual transaction; "there is nothing they can do." Finally, the condom, that technology that both *Wazungu* and African medical authorities agree is the best way to prevent HIV, did not offer security or certainty in the face of this enormous crisis. The conclusion that I drew from how the nurses defined these problems was that "European" research and development projects that put the responsibility of stopping AIDS on African women were for the nurses at best misguided and at worst very dangerous.

The nurses' perspectives helped me see the contradiction that is the focus of this book. Since almost the start of the AIDS pandemic, there has been evidence that the majority of the world's women are put at greatest risk of HIV infection because they live, have sex, and get pregnant in contexts that continually affirm the existence of an exclusively masculine right to act on individual sexual desire without regard to the desires, needs, or well-being of partner, child, or community. In an apparent paradox, however, internationally funded and nationally sanctioned interventions to stop the spread of HIV have focused almost exclusively on the sexual and reproductive behaviors of the working-class and poor women of color around the world who are least able to challenge such constructions of masculine sexuality and the material inequalities that support it. *Local Women, Global Science* represents my efforts to explain the origins, the scientific elaboration, and the implementation of this fundamental and dangerous contradiction.

Hints that this contradiction existed and that it posed enormous challenges in Nairobi's clinics came from many of the stories I was told by nurses and from the interactions I witnessed between nurses and researchers on the one hand and nurses and patients on the other. I heard repeatedly about "irresponsible African men" who "go around" (that is, sleep around) and callously bring home infection after infection to their wives. Nurses told me and their female patients that these men were likely to beat up a wife who asked them to get treated or use a condom. The nurses gave patients the antibiotics that an HIV/STD research and control project, which was staffed and funded by Europeans, brought to their clinics. Frequently, however, the nurses did not actually give condoms to their female patients, suggest ways women might negotiate with their partners for safer sex, or encourage women with STDs or symptoms of HIV infection to bring their male sexual partners for treatment. The nurses never criticized the project to stop HIV. They did not perceive themselves to be resisting, reframing, or reinterpreting health policy or medical protocol. They were convinced, however, that there was very little chance that the women who came to them for help could ever get a man to use a condom or otherwise change his sexual behavior.

The nurses were not alone in their views, nor was their sense of women's position unsubstantiated. By the early 1990s, ethnographic studies had demonstrated that although many women know that their husband or partner is having sex with other women, they do not feel entitled to demand that he use a condom. We had also learned that many women fear being beaten or abandoned if they suggest to their partner that he stop seeing other women or even that he use a condom. A number of feminist scholars have written about the multiple victimization of many of the world's poorest women by HIV, by male sexual domination and promiscuity, and by the economic conditions that make it impossible for women to leave the men who put them at risk.[9]

These studies also suggest that most of the women at highest risk of infection expect, want, and often are required to become pregnant. For many women living in the countries hardest hit by AIDS, pregnancy and motherhood are the key to enjoying some privilege in their communities. Many poor women also depend on their adult children for economic and emotional support, particularly during periods of crisis (Hartmann 1995; Baylies 2000). By the early 1990s, HIV-positive women, their noninfected advocates, and feminist researchers from many different countries were arguing that until there was a female-controlled method of protecting ourselves from HIV transmission during heterosexual intercourse and a convenient and affordable way to get pregnant without at the same time getting infected, the relative ability or inability of women to get their men to use condoms would have a decisive impact on the extent and shape of the epidemic.

Feminist research, as well as feminist political movements, however, demand that we question claims that any woman or group of women is ever completely powerless. Studies of sexual practices from Kenya, elsewhere in sub-Saharan Africa, and in many other parts of the world demonstrate that women are never simply heterosexual men's victims or pawns.[10] However subtly at times and in spite of the risks, women constantly negotiate when, where, how, and with whom they will or will not have sex. Nairobi's nurses themselves frequently commented on the determination of their patients to get STD treatment and to use contraceptives even when expressly, sometimes violently, forbidden to do so by husbands or partners.[11]

Why, then, did the nurses at Casino and Bestlands view their female patients as sexual victims and why did they act on that view in the face of researchers' expectations that the nurses would do otherwise? I began to ask this question about midway through my research on the construction of "the woman problem" in international AIDS policy discourse. I had finished interviewing state officials and international AIDS policymakers and reading hundreds of policy documents and medical reports. I was just beginning the "local" part of my study—with almost no idea of what I was looking for or what I would see—by getting to know the nurses working at Casino, which was "AIDS research central" in Nairobi at the time. What I saw and heard suggested to me that quite unconsciously the nurses were *selectively* accepting and rejecting aspects of the AIDS-control project that the Kenyan state, the World Health Organization's (WHO) Global Programme on AIDS (GPA), and a team of foreign medical researchers had together imposed on their clinics.

Janet and her co-workers at Casino and Sister Kiroro and her staff at Bestlands justified their decisions about condoms and contact tracing by asserting that they knew without asking that their female patients were unable or unwilling to comply with what the nurses perceived to be "European" expectations about heterosexual negotiation. Moreover, the nurses were certain that they could do nothing to change "African" women's position. And if they could not, they suggested, nobody could. Masculine sexual dominance and what they typically referred to as men's irresponsibility were natural to Kenyan men, they told me. This dominance predated AIDS and was both fixed and unstoppable.

Other components of the control strategy, however, were not problematic at all. The nurses had no difficulty agreeing to carry out project demands that they classify symptoms in the very precise way dictated by a treatment "algorithm" invented entirely by *Wazungu* researchers. These demands added an enormous burden to the already overworked and underpaid nurses by increasing their paperwork as well as the time it took them to diagnose and counsel women. The nurses were forced to reorganize (and sometimes reorganize again) their daily work routines in order to comply. Implementing these requirements also made the clinics, and by extension the nurses, dependent on the very limited drugs, technology, supplies, and training provided exclusively by the development agencies, universities, and pharmaceutical companies that the *Wazungu* represented. The nurses were constantly aware that they could stop getting these resources any day if the researchers became unhappy with or uninterested in their clinics. Nevertheless, they apparently eagerly took on the burden of the extra work, the tension of being watched and evaluated by the *Wazungu,* and the difficulties of translating to their patients what they were doing, why it was important, and what it had to do with AIDS.

To a woman, the nurses agreed that they felt "lucky" to have the researchers and the projects in their clinic. Their national government was beset by economic and political crises and was impoverished by a combination of internal corruption, declining foreign investment and terms of trade in the global market, and the withdrawal of economic assistance by donor countries fed up with Kenya's unwillingness to restructure its economy and no longer worried that Kenya might fall to the communists, a "problem" resolved by the end of the Cold War.[12] The state had stopped providing drugs and other essential medical supplies to public clinics all over the country—first in rural areas and finally in downtown Nairobi itself. The *Wazungu* stepped in, giving the staff of clinics that were "lucky" enough to be included in their research and implementation projects something to do when patients came in to see them. The nurses' praise of the project and those funding it made their unwillingness to carry out key components of the project more visible and exposed the dangerous contradictions underlying these policies.

This book emerged out of my effort to reanalyze national and international AIDS policy and the scientific research on which it was based from where I sat in clinic rooms listening to conversations between nurses and patients. It struck me that by understanding how nurses interpreted, translated, and negotiated the demands that this project and the discourses of "AIDS crisis" more generally placed on them, I might "see" at least part of why efforts to control AIDS had thus far largely failed. Perhaps these nurses and their experiences could in some way begin to explain why the nearly twenty years of debate, scientific research, and technological advancement in the service of AIDS control as well as decades of efforts to reduce the spread of other more-treatable and better-understood STDs had not had much impact on sexual practices.

Nurses are predominantly female the world over. They are also among the workers most directly and intimately involved in tying women's bodies, particularly those of working-class and poor women, to state institutions and state control. Nevertheless, astonishingly few feminist social scientists have taken nurses seriously as social actors worthy of study, particularly in Third World contexts. Those who have studied nurses as social, economic, and political agents argue, based on quite different studies, that nurses occupy a critical position brokering relationships between policymakers, medical scientists, financers of health care, public perceptions of women and diseases, and patients.[13] Yet no social scientist concerned about AIDS in Africa has bothered to talk to nurses about the crisis there. In the face of such silence, I came to believe that nurses might teach us a great deal about how "globalization" actually operates on and in the everyday locations and practices of the state.

It is critical to note that this study is also limited by my choice to focus on nurses and, to a lesser extent, on the North American and European researchers for whom they worked. My ethnographic material comes from my effort to take the standpoint of some nurses at a specific moment in time with respect to the AIDS crisis and foreign interventions in it. By focusing on the practices and views of a small group of middle-class, formally educated nurses, I chose not to investigate the relative agency or victimization or the actual sexual desires, needs, or practices of working-class women in Nairobi. The perceptions of heterosexuality, gender, race, and class that I analyze here are my interpretations of the ways that nurses working in two of Nairobi's most important clinics during the early 1990s perceived themselves, their position in a global crisis, and their patients. I do not claim that their perceptions of women's behaviors and needs were "correct" in any way. Indeed, part of my argument is that the nurses' assumptions that working-class women are virtually powerless in heterosexual relationships form an important part of the explanation for why the clinics have had relatively little effect on the epidemic.

Wamuuchi, Janet, Sister Kiroro, and their co-workers perform much of the work required by the AIDS research and development project I studied in Kenya. It falls mainly to middle-class African women who have been trained in medicine for anywhere from two to six years to bring scientific knowledge and health technology to bear on the treatment and counseling of Kenyan women. They are also responsible for transforming Kenyan women into cooperative subjects for HIV/AIDS research. Nonetheless, none of the enormous number of studies of HIV in Africa has considered the perspectives of nurses to be an important influence on how people understand or cope with the epidemic. No study has attempted to understand AIDS, whether as a local problem or as a transnational phenomenon, from the position of African nurses. It is safe to say, in fact, that the nurses who do so much of the work involved in bringing the science, policy, and technology of HIV/AIDS to individuals at risk in Africa and delivering most of the data we have about heterosexual AIDS have been rendered invisible by the design, conduct, and publication of that research.

To make the nurses and their work visible requires that we see how their everyday work at Bestlands and Casino is simultaneously "local" and "global." Before I can explain how this can be so, we must take a closer look at the perhaps too widely used and certainly too rarely defined terms of this apparent opposition. There has been a great deal of debate crossing many disciplines about what global and local mean and to what, if any, "real world" places, events, or relationships they refer. A thorough engagement with these debates is beyond the scope of this book. The discussions have, however, generated several insights that are especially relevant to those who employ ethnographic methods to understand some of the dynamics of a "global" crisis.

Just who, what, or where is the global? How does the concept of the global help us make sense of the experiences of nurses such as Janet and Wamuuchi? The many and often-interesting debates that are taking place over the term suggest that if the concept is to be useful at all it must be specified in relation to a particular moment or set of relationships (Massey 1994; Gupta 1998; Burawoy 2000a). "Global" is not, in short, a global (or universal) concept. I use the term in two different but related ways. First, it is my shorthand for specific processes, such as the spread of HIV, structural adjustment programs, the most labor-intensive parts of textile manufacturing, and tourism, that cannot be explained without reference to people, organizations, economic trends, or conflicts that transcend traditional national and regional boundaries. Likewise, the many and various problems created by these processes cannot be addressed without understanding their global dimensions. For example, the significant increases in maternal and infant mortality and in infectious diseases such as tuberculosis and hepatitis reported by a number of sub-Saharan African countries appear to be an indirect effect of structural adjustment programs imposed by transnational organizations in the name of promoting global trade (Wakhweya 1995). Such programs have increased income inequality while drastically reducing the availability of subsidies and social services (Hoogvelt 2001).

Another, related, use of the term global is as a way to identify, explain, and even resolve problems shared by people living in different parts of the world. The editor of the British medical journal *The Lancet* used the notion of global in this way when discussing debates over how to prevent the spread of HIV among intravenous drug users and their partners:

> The commonality in this respect [the experience of HIV-related discrimination] of homosexuals in Iran, intravenous drug abusers in New York, and Nepalese women with "India disease" as a result of cross-border prostitution is readily apparent. Yet why should drug users in Bangkok be able to hold down steady jobs and be part of mainstream society whereas their counterparts in the USA who seek clean syringes are promptly imprisoned? There, surely, is one small example of how rational global thinking to frame intravenous drug use as a public health and not a moral issue might influence local strategy. (1993, 1625)

The WHO's creation of a "global" program to stop AIDS was premised on this expectation that unified or standardized (rationalized) health policies could address related problems across the world's large variety of local experiences and identities.

I also follow the ethnographic practice of using "native" terminology in the same way that the "natives," here international and national AIDS bureaucrats, do. In interviews and on paper, key actors described

HIV/AIDS as a global disease and a global crisis. This was especially common in the hallways, meetings, and documents of the WHO's AIDS program, which has called itself global since 1988. Rather than containing any inherent, consistent, or fixed meaning, the adjective served as an important linguistic tool in this community. WHO officials' use (never accompanied by a definition) of the term global to describe the problem of AIDS expressed the organization's initial interest in being seen by governments, researchers, and activists as the only organization capable of transcending the national and local politics that the WHO's leaders believed to be obstacles to prevention and control.

To define a crisis as global is to assert that the problem is immediate and urgent and that it should be everyone's top priority. The term reflected the WHO's early determination to get immediate attention and money from wealthy countries. The adjective also frightens; it suggests that everyone is under threat. The spread of HIV in one country puts every country, and therefore every person, in the world at risk. Finally, the WHO's Global Programme on AIDS was set apart from the organization's other programs in the name of global crisis. Neither a "world" nor an "international" program, the GPA was special. Its staff solicited money directly from donor countries, and funding, hiring, and policy-making bypassed the bureaucratic red tape through which other units had to go. Unlike the directors of the WHO's other departments, who were expected to behave apolitically and objectively, the heads of the AIDS program were able to criticize recalcitrant national governments openly and often quite undiplomatically. At the WHO, then, the "global" signified that which was new, distinct, unusual, powerful, and urgent, adjectives that might be used to describe AIDS itself.

What or where, then, is the "local," that entity commonly used to describe whatever the global is not? A number of scholars have argued that ever since humans began migrating, there has not been an empirical distinction between that which is local and that which is not. Doreen Massey (1994), Michael Burawoy (2000a; 2000b), Aihwa Ong (1987; 1999), and Saskia Sassen (1998), to name just a few, have suggested that the "global" can only be "seen" or analyzed from within local subjectivities, spaces, relationships, and discourses. As important, they have pointed out that what appears to be local is never independent from or knowable without reference to processes originating outside it and beyond its control. It may be useful methodologically, even necessary, to analyze events, places, people, and discourses as if they are local. Nevertheless, these scholars argue, such analyses assume boundaries that are illusory.

Feminist geographer Doreen Massey has been particularly clear about the need to rethink what we mean by the local. She argues that those who think they can see a clear distinction and can therefore identify a set of things that are purely "local" (or "global") are living a powerful fantasy. The fantasy is that one has or could have a "home," a truly local space that is safe from external forces and events over which, it seems, individuals have no control. Massey points out that although many observers like to argue that the loss of such a space is a recent phenomenon, in fact colonized people everywhere have for centuries been prohibited from experiencing even the illusion of pure "locality."[14] Colonized and colonizing women alike, moreover, have never been guaranteed safety or control within their homes. Like colonization, the virtual universality of domestic violence demonstrates that this notion of the local in reality describes the experience of very few of the world's people.

In every locale—a clinic in Nairobi, a United Nations (UN) office in Geneva, a medical laboratory in Manitoba—people's lives are shaped by processes, information, and technology originating elsewhere and by relationships with both known and unknown people living their lives in distant places. Every process defined as global is both generated and experienced in specific, if complex and often heavily guarded, local spaces and moments. One unusually clear example of the importance of location to the production of the global is the 2002 meeting of the World Trade Organization (WTO) held in Doha, the capital of Qatar. The selection of this city at this time as the site for the controversial meetings of the organization in charge of global trade and the distribution of the profits and the costs resulting from it had an important effect. Qatari laws prohibiting public assembly and free speech locally enabled the WTO to avoid facing direct challenges from AIDS and anti-globalization activists who have been mobilizing all over the world. Deliberations about forcing countries to obey multinational pharmaceutical corporations' patents on AIDS treatments, for example, were kept out of the public, that is, the global, eye. We visit these and other discussions of the AIDS drug conflict in the final chapter.

Different locales and the people in them, are not, however, equally powerful, equally able to see, control, or move out of the relationships and decisions that affect their everyday lives. As Massey insists, to understand the local and global as always already existing within each other is not to collapse or ignore the enormous inequalities between different locales and the people within them. Massey's aim is to make visible the way that the inequalities of capitalism, which are always reproduced in local settings such as board rooms, factory floors, and WTO meetings, have been creating massive inequalities between geographic regions during and since the periods of official European and

American imperialism. Capitalism has, she and other feminists remind us, relied on and intensified both gender and racial inequalities in the production of geographic inequality.[15]

Ethnographies are commonly considered useful only for studying phenomena that have or seem to have clear and knowable boundaries—that are, therefore, "local." According to many scholars (including both those who do ethnographies and those who do not), the conclusions drawn from ethnographic research are valid only for a specific place, people, and time.[16] Recent challenges to the notion that the local is the antithesis of (and obscures) "the global," therefore, are crucial for those of us who wish to defend the ethnographic method as a tool for making visible crucial dimensions of crises such as the spread of HIV (Burawoy 2000b).

A global ethnography of the HIV/AIDS crisis, then, has to focus on how the crisis has been fueled by transnational migration, international tourism, and the production and export of military technology, war, and refugees. It has to insist that women and men in one part of the world experience risk and disease the way they do partly because of how the causes, parameters, and solutions of these crises are defined by researchers, agencies, governments, and corporations that are located or headquartered elsewhere. Such a study must recognize that apparently local levels and outcomes of HIV infection and the shape of national or community efforts to resist it are determined by relationships between people who have never met, between people who never would have met if the crisis had not brought them together, and even between people who belong to different historical moments. Simultaneously, the global ethnographer must understand how sexual, material, and ideological relationships between members of the same family, village, neighborhood, or nation determine the spread of infection and the interpretations of the disease.

The legacy of ethnography as the explication only of the "local" has not been erased, however. Less than twenty years ago, my undergraduate anthropology professors trained me to learn and celebrate the ethnographic method because it generated "local," "concrete," and "relative" (that is, noncomparable) knowledge about people and things that had been strange to me. In a graduate seminar on the anthropology of gender and work, Ann Stoler turned this way of seeing upside down for me. When I looked back over the ethnographic fieldnotes that I took during this study and in earlier research, however, I realized that like other ethnographers, I remain influenced by the traditional view of the method. Despite my consistent interest in doing a study of "transnational AIDS," I often found that the questions I asked or the ways I described things that I saw (and the things that I chose to see) assumed the existence of some kind of temporal and geographic fixity. Sometimes I assumed that what I was told or what I saw existed in precisely the same way before I came along and would continue to exist in that way after I left. In the chapters that follow, I try to call attention to how such assumptions might have affected what I learned from Nairobi's nurses. Of course, I am sure that I cannot see all the ways or moments in which I imposed this assumption on "my field."

This study takes as its starting point the experiences of nurses in an underresourced public clinic in the capital city of a crisis-ridden country on the world's poorest continent. Nurses confront policies based on revived and revamped imperial views of venereal disease that have been translated first into contracts for donor-country assistance by senior international and national bureaucrats and second into science and medical care by foreign researchers and local health care workers. The location is Nairobi, the East African city built for Europeans in the middle of land that appeared to the British to belong to no one. The history of European settlement and the making of an "African" Nairobi—a process of segregation partially organized and justified by British perceptions that Africans "harbored" venereal diseases—is a critical part of this global/local story. I describe a three-year period during which *Wazungu* medical researchers and publicly employed nurses turned mostly female patients in two clinics into the objects of a large, multinationally funded, research-oriented health development project. This project has been most authoritatively presented to certain audiences in the world beyond Nairobi in more than 400 scientific reports about STDs, including HIV/AIDS, among prostitutes, men, and mothers living with HIV or living at risk in the city. *Local Women, Global Science* offers an alternative representation of these years that takes into account Nairobi's past and current political economy and the experiences of women nurses struggling to cope with the sexist and racist organization of health care for the poor in the time of AIDS.

As a global ethnography, this study looks beyond the nurses, Nairobi, and the early 1990s. I suggest that understanding what happened in Nairobi and internationally leading up to and during the early 1990s will help us understand the apparently quite different debates taking place today over AIDS in Africa and transnationally. Kenyans, Ugandans, and South Africans with HIV; U.S., British, French, and South African AIDS activists; executives of multinational pharmaceutical companies; African and Euro-American medical researchers; and international health, development, and trade organizations are all embroiled in debates over who deserves treatment and on whom such treatments should be tested.

Several apparently unconnected events that took place between 1992 and 1995 contributed to the emergence of these latest debates. At the start of the decade, a new regime at the WHO proclaimed that women in the so-called developing countries were in the best position of all to care for the infected and to prevent the further spread of the disease. Shortly after that, the same agency announced that it was (paradoxically) drastically downsizing its AIDS intervention efforts in sub-Saharan Africa. Soon after this, in 1994, a clinical trial conducted on HIV-positive pregnant women in the United States demonstrated that the drug azidothymidine (AZT) significantly reduced the probability that they would transmit their infections to their babies (Connor et al. 1994). During the years this trial ran, the European and North American researchers in Nairobi expanded their HIV/STD project beyond its initial focus on prostitutes; they took their work to clinics such as Bestlands that are devoted mainly to providing maternal and child health care and birth control. Meanwhile, Kenya's ruling party was reeling from having very nearly lost its 30-year control of the state. Collectively, these events of the early 1990s helped to bring us to the situation we face at the start of the new millennium: an ethical, medical, economic, and political crisis that hurts first and foremost the world's working-class and poor women but that ultimately affects us all.

Understanding Kenya's HIV epidemic requires that we be aware of the relations of class and gender inequality that determine who has been and will be the most vulnerable to infection and the least able to find information or treatment. During the late 1980s, it seemed that everyone was at risk, regardless of income or status. There was a great deal of concern about the impact AIDS would have on Kenya's tiny middle and ruling classes. Development experts were warning state elites that they, as well as teachers, policemen, military personnel, and health care workers, would be devastated (Panos 1989 and 1990; Mann, Tarantola, and Netter 1992). A handful of people from elite families in other African countries began "coming out" as HIV positive. There were many rumors that certain high-level politicians and civil servants in Kenya were infected. The daily newspapers reported that middle-class or aspiring college women were put at risk by older, rich "sugar daddies" in order to get school fees and clothing. Several observers warned of the "vacuum" of power likely to result from the unchecked spread of HIV.

In Kenya, as in other parts of the world, however, it soon became apparent that the distribution of risk was not equal. The people who were most vulnerable to infection (and to early death) were those whose survival was highly uncertain or so dependent on the incomes or desires of others that they could not afford to protect themselves. Landless women and men who have been forced to migrate and who face a limited set of ways to generate income are now at the greatest risk of becoming infected, of having no treatment, and of dying. The distribution of HIV infection, like the distribution of most debilitating illnesses, can be understood only with reference to the distribution of wealth and the bodily autonomy that accompanies it. In Kenya, as elsewhere, gender and class are the main forces shaping that distribution.

Kenya has one of the subcontinent's, and one of the world's, most unequal distributions of income and land. According to a recent and remarkable study by Mwangi wa Gîthînjî (2000), the wealthiest 10 percent of the rural population receives nearly 65 percent of rural wealth. The poorer half of rural Kenyans receive less than 9 percent of that wealth (39). Urban wealth is somewhat more evenly distributed; in the cities the richest 10 percent receive about half of the total urban income. The bottom 50 percent of city-dwellers receive 17 percent (39). The current distribution of wealth in Kenya runs remarkably parallel to the distribution of land under colonial rule; only the skin color has changed. The highest incomes go to the small number of large land-owners in what was once called the "white highlands," the fertile and temperate area just north of Nairobi. During colonial rule, the "highlands" were reserved by Britain for white growers of tea and coffee. Subsequently, the Kenyan state granted the land vacated by settlers at independence to politically important Kenyan families. Gîthînjî calculates that the income gap between the rich and the poor in this region is the largest in the country. The poorest people in the highlands are the children of those whom the settlers kicked off the land and transformed into agricultural laborers and urban migrants.

The legacy of colonialism and the post-independence state's commitment to essentially unbridled capitalist accumulation are also quite visible in the organization of gender relations in Kenya. The colonial government was often brutally insensitive to the fact that rural Kenyan women performed the bulk of subsistence agricultural production and to the extremely unequal distribution of what few economic benefits there were to be had for Kenyans living in a settler colony. Settlers preferred to have "native" men as their domestic and agricultural employees. African women were virtually invisible to the settlers, although they often (illegally) lived and worked on the plantations alongside their husbands and fathers (Stichter 1985). The state wanted to keep African women out of the towns and cities, in part to ensure that male workers did not become permanent residents, in part because they knew that rural women grew the food crops that helped keep male wages low, and in part to appease rural patriarchs (Stichter 1985; White 1990).

Independent Kenya's first president, Jomo Kenyatta, had no interest in redressing the gender inequalities produced at the intersection of colonial and precolonial social and economic organization. He believed that women contributed little to the economy (Aubrey 1997). His somewhat successful (and internationally acclaimed) efforts to get rural communities to fund and build their own health and education facilities, however, relied heavily on, and greatly increased, women's unpaid, unrecognized labor (Aubrey 1997). President Daniel arap Moi continued Kenyatta's basic neglect of women's issues. Lisa Aubrey comments that "beyond broad statements of recognition and praise for compliant women and the consequent 'good' intentions of government to support women, there is very little substantive policy or genuine commitment to assist women" (66). Government spending in Kenya has clearly demonstrated that women's programs are an extremely low priority. Between 1978 and 1982, 0.1 percent of government spending went to women's programs (67). Astonishingly, particularly given that in 1985 the third UN Conference on Women was held in Nairobi and brought enormous (if temporary) international attention to the conditions under which many East African women live, this percentage has actually decreased since then (67).

Unofficial sexism is part of the everyday practice of the Kenyan state. Until very recently, the government refused to address even rhetorically the very high rates of rape, domestic abuse, and deaths due to botched abortions that Kenyan women experience. The most visible women's organization, Maendeleo ya Wanawake (MyWO), has suffered both government repression and cooptation; except in rare instances, it has failed to represent poor and working women in either rural or urban areas (Aubrey 1997; Nzomo 1997). Although in recent years it has managed to shake itself free of total control by the ruling party, MyWO is nonetheless still perceived to be state-owned and guided by the interests of elite women. Members of more radical and grassroots women's organizations as well as women union members, sex workers, and outspoken widows of the state's political enemies have repeatedly been harassed, imprisoned, tortured, made into objects of ridicule, and simply ignored.

Of course, this political inequality has its economic analog. In the cities, women earn between 42 and 69 percent of men's earnings and spend many fewer of their working hours in paid employment. During the 1990s, the approximately 17 percent of urban households that were headed by women received less than half the income received by households headed by men. The gap is even wider in the rural areas (Gîthînjî 2000, 80). In the following chapters, I will discuss what it means in such a context to talk about "empowering" women in the fight against HIV/AIDS.

During the winter and spring of 1993, when I was visiting the clinics, the Kenyan people confronted enormous political and economic uncertainty. In December of 1992, Kenya held its first multiparty presidential and parliamentary elections in twenty-eight years. Despite several years of political excitement and energetic organizing by their opponents, the president and the ruling party, the Kenya African National Union (KANU), won again. But the new government was no longer entirely under Moi's control; the pre-election organizing had created new spaces for dissent both inside and outside the state (Huband 2001; Holmquist and Ford 1994). It was not yet clear, however, what and who would fill those spaces or if, somehow, KANU would find a way to close them again. As part of his campaign to stay in power and to end what was referred to as multipartyism,[17] Moi's supporters fomented a civil war in central Kenya (Huband 2001). Meanwhile, Moi's repeated failures to implement the structural adjustment programs that were imposed and reimposed on the country by the International Monetary Fund had resulted in the canceling of monetary aid and loans from the multilateral and bilateral agencies supported by North American and Western European governments (Wrong 1995). Newspaper and radio reports showcasing Moi's attempts to blame "western imperialism" for the country's increasingly severe economic crisis contributed to an atmosphere of tension, confusion, fear, and uncertainty in the city.

Although never discussed openly by any party during the elections, the rapidly growing epidemic of HIV infection played no small role in creating and perpetuating these tensions. Kenya was one of the first countries both to attract North American and Western European AIDS researchers and to be blamed for spreading the virus to the rest of the world. The government has periodically been a very vocal participant in some of the most contentious international fights over the pandemic.

When I arrived in Nairobi in 1992, the United States Agency for International Development (USAID) had just completed a survey indicating that 11 percent of Nairobi's population was infected with HIV.[18] More ominously, the report stated that prevalence among the city's women was slightly higher than that among men and was increasing more rapidly (USAID 1991). Eighty percent of Nairobi women identified as prostitutes were infected (Plummer et al. 1994). As figure 1.1 shows, rates of infection among pregnant women coming to public clinics increased from 0 percent in 1985 to as high as 17 percent in some parts of the city (USAID 1991). The prevalence of infection among pregnant women is commonly considered to be a good indicator of infection levels among the so-called general population. Figure 1.2 indicates a parallel rate of increase in HIV infection among men who had been diagnosed with an STD associated with HIV. Levels of prevalence among these men, however, were consistently much higher than among pregnant women. Evidence was also emerging that among the city's adolescents, women were getting infected at a younger age and at faster rates than men (Glynn et al. 2001). Unfortunately, USAID followed the U.S. practice of not collecting data comparing prevalence rates among the rich and poor. The 11 percent estimate was calculated on the basis of reported cases of AIDS and the occasional HIV prevalence study. Because they came from public hospitals and clinics, these data hid from view most HIV infections among the wealthy, who would have gone to private doctors. To date, there is no unequivocal evidence that low-income Kenyans are more likely to be infected than those with higher incomes.

Kenya's official responses to the first reports of cases of AIDS in East Africa seemed contradictory. On the one hand, the minister of health called a meeting of national and expatriate scientists and representatives of the WHO to discuss the disease and establish diagnostic and reporting guidelines that Kenya's doctors would be required to follow. Kenya was comparatively quick to create a national AIDS committee and an AIDS-control plan, establish a blood-screening program, introduce information about AIDS into health care worker training curricula, put up "stop AIDS" posters, and broadcast a radio program providing basic information about HIV in most of the country's major languages.

At the same time, however, President Moi was publicly silent on the issue, except when he was denying that AIDS posed an important threat. In the same month that the minister of health was mobilizing experts and information, the minister of tourism officially denied that AIDS existed in the country. President Moi had several thousand copies of an issue of the *International Herald Tribune* confiscated because it reported that British naval troops were passing up their usual shore leave in Mombasa due to AIDS. Even after it became impossible to deny that HIV was a problem, the Kenyan government continued to frustrate domestic and foreign AIDS experts as well as people living with the disease (Fortin 1987; 1990). Throughout the 1990s, President Moi was unwilling to speak out about AIDS or safer sex, publicize accurate statistics on the spread of the virus, create a budget dedicated to AIDS-control, protect stigmatized groups, or acknowledge the existence or struggles of Kenyans living with AIDS. When Jonathan Mann, the first

Percent of
Pregnant Women
Attending Clinics

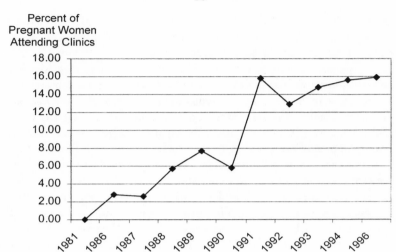

Source: U.S. Census Bureau 2002.

Figure 1.1 HIV Prevalence in Pregnant Women Attending Public Antenatal
Clinics, Nairobi, 1981–1996 (percent)

director of the WHO's GPA, referred in his frequent speeches to a
"lack of political will" to confront the crisis among African governments, there was little doubt that he was speaking to and about Kenya,
among other countries.

Most of these problems were not unique to Kenya. Although Uganda
responded quickly and with much-better-funded, more explicit and aggressive, and more nuanced HIV interventions, Tanzania's efforts were
thwarted by a severe economic crisis like that faced by Kenya. The governments of Malawi, Zimbabwe, Zambia, and, more recently, South Africa have been reluctant either to discuss or confront the disease.

Moreover, from virtually the beginning of the epidemic, many governments in sub-Saharan Africa, North America, Europe, and Asia
joined Kenya in making low-income women of color the primary targets
of HIV-control measures. Although scientists and policymakers have
very recently begun to address the role of heterosexual men in spreading HIV,[19] the tendency to blame women for reproducing the crisis and
to target them with interventions that often do not respond to their desires, needs, or capacities continues almost everywhere during the third
decade of the pandemic. By focusing on the processes involved in making and reproducing this disastrous construction of women in Nairobi,

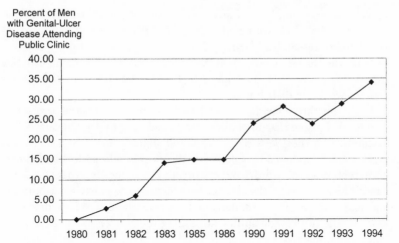

Source: U.S. Census Bureau 2002.

Figure 1.2 HIV Prevalence in Male STD Patients Diagnosed with Genital-Ulcer Disease, Nairobi Special Treatment Clinic, 1980–1996 (percent)

this book calls attention to the serious contradictions and very real dangers of these transnational trends and argues for an alternative approach that supports women's own efforts to mobilize for political and economic power.

Each of the following chapters visits a different locale, beginning in Nairobi's special clinic for sexually transmitted disease. Chapter 2 locates the reader in the middle of Kenya's AIDS crisis and in the middle of downtown Nairobi by describing Casino, Kenya's first STD clinic and the base for much of the early research on AIDS in the country. I describe the intersections of colonial, global, and local relations in the reproduction of this important "glocality" in the world's AIDS crisis. I trace the influences of racist and gendered colonial medical science and policy on current understandings of sexuality and disease in the African city.

In chapter 3, I summarize the Kenyan government's response to HIV/AIDS during the first decade of the crisis by focusing on two processes: one, the unraveling of the national political economy and the response of international financial organizations and foreign donors, and two, the often-hostile negotiations over "AIDS policy" between the WHO's GPA and Kenya's Ministry of Health. As Kenya's political and economic crises made its health crisis even worse, and as rates of HIV prevalence rose rapidly in Nairobi and other cities, national and international AIDS officials wrangled over limited resources and policy priorities. Foreign researchers bearing drugs, information, and other supplies became the de facto policymakers in local urban clinics. The public nurses on whom they depended, in turn, determined how these resources would be distributed.

I take up the biomedical foundation of the HIV-control project in chapter 4. I argue that to explain the spread of HIV in Nairobi, AIDS researchers in the 1980s resurrected and slightly reworked a racist and sexist model developed by colonial medical experts to understand apparently high rates of syphilis and gonorrhea among newly urbanized Kenyans. The objective of the chapter is to identify the scientific elaboration and justification of the fundamental contradiction of AIDS discourse that put the full responsibility for ending the pandemic on African urban women.

In chapter 5, the story returns to the clinic level. This chapter demonstrates the complexity and importance of nurses' responses to HIV and the crisis in heterosexuality to which the virus's continued spread points. The chapter describes the everyday worklife of nurses in a clinic historically devoted to promoting the use of contraceptives to women and now transformed into a "demonstration site" for a foreign-funded project to prevent HIV infection in pregnant women. I argue that nurses daily produce policy by brokering and selectively translating relationships among biomedicine and development; donors and the state; past and present economic, political, and sexual relations; and experts and patients. In this process, nurses actively interpret, challenge, and reframe "expert" knowledge about HIV and African women. On the local level, therefore, policy in the form of everyday institutional practices reflects not only tensions and accommodations between the national and the international but also the nurses' own class, race, and gender interests.

By way of moving beyond the previous chapters' critique of what has already happened in Kenya, chapter 6 discusses the current international fight over who should get what HIV drugs, when, and at what financial and ethical costs. I situate Kenya's crisis within the global struggle over the profits and power to be gained by controlling the definition of HIV and of its treatment. The chapter briefly takes up the case of South Africa, currently the most visible, and internally divided, of the sub-Saharan African countries pressuring multinational pharmaceutical companies to make HIV drugs affordable, particularly to infected pregnant women. The book concludes by reflecting on the ways that women's varying experiences as mothers can and must be made a productive basis for women's (and potentially men's) political organizing in response to the deadly gender, race, and national inequalities that HIV is exposing. Although the roles of scientific object and of patient define mothers as passive, nurses' constructions open up toward more active, indeed political, framings of maternal experiences. I suggest that nurses and their women patients can work together both inside and outside the clinic to redefine their collective sexual and health needs and to demand from state and international agencies that these needs be met.

Two

Nairobi's Casino
Colonizing AIDS in the Urban Clinic

The Special Treatment Clinic popularly known as Casino is not easy to find. Not, that is, if you are a young white woman wandering solo in Nairobi's downtown. To get there from where I was living near the Ministry of Health, one literally has to descend into the center of town and pass through the central area where tourists mingle in hotel cafés, curio shops, and expensive Indian restaurants; where Kenyan tour guides hustle business for their safari companies; and where the for-tourists-only taxis stand. This place is familiar and "safe" for a white woman; I blend in perfectly. But to find the clinic, one has to go out of and behind this space. In fact, just behind and a bit to the west of the enormous Nairobi Hilton is an area where few tourists go, just a few steps but a whole world away from the part of town Kenya offers to most visitors. This is an area with far too much "local color" for the typical holiday-maker on safari.

"Be careful down there." "Don't go alone." "Take a taxi to the clinic." I was often warned in phrases such as these by friends, Kenyan and *Wazungu* alike, when they learned of my research plans.[1] In conversations with clinic staff, I learned that many of them, especially the middle-class women, felt unsafe coming to work; several described the neighborhood as a "very risky" place. Armed guards were always leaning against the doors of the clinic, quite visible to all who passed. But who or what was being protected? Who or what was the enemy? The clinic's immediate neighbors were mostly small shops from which Kenyan and Asian men sold bootlegged music cassettes. The old Casino Theatre around the corner, which lent its name to the clinic, showed outdated blockbusters from both Hollywood and Bollywood, the source of very popular South Asian melodramas. I had been in parts of the city where people appeared to be much more desperately poor and where I had actually seen muggings and a variety of other dangerous and illegal activities. Casino's neighborhood seemed serene by comparison. After I had spent a few weeks at the clinic, it started to become clear that the main "danger" Casino represented lay in the fact that it was still a monument to beliefs held by Kenya's colonizers and inherited by members of the postcolonial civil service. These beliefs concerned the various supposed risks that having Africans in a "white" city posed.

Casino's location was determined well before its doors opened in the early 1950s. In 1899, when the builders of the Kenya-Uganda Railroad (KUR) and the fledgling colonial government selected Nairobi as their respective headquarters, they put into effect a racialized urban planning policy. Like many cities throughout the empire, Nairobi was entirely invented by the colonizers. Where East Africa's largest city now stands, there was only open grassland and swamp, "uninhabited" to British eyes blind to the migration patterns of the pastoralist Maasai in the region (Obudho and Aduwo 1992, 50). Nairobi grew quickly into a city rigidly segregated by race. Europeans immediately settled in the cool and fertile hills west of the railroad and the administrative buildings. Asians were restricted to the less-appealing areas north of the center (Cooper 1983; Obudho and Aduwo 1992). Until 1923, there was no official area for Africans. In that year, the government created Pangani, a housing estate to the east of the city center that became Nairobi's most famous "African location," later known as Pumwani. It is on the very edge of Pumwani, where the neighborhood bumps into the administrative and tourist center, that Casino stands.

Nairobi appealed to the Europeans in large part for health reasons. Its hills were free of malaria and its river promised a stable and clean water supply. Urban planning reflected Europeans' determination to keep the members of their community healthy (Kurtz 1998, 77). According to Obudho and Aduwo (1992), overcrowding, poor drainage in the swampy slums, and the malnutrition resulting from low wages, all products of European settlement and racism, soon created the very health problems that Europeans had expected to avoid in Nairobi. Malaria, plague, pneumonia, and tuberculosis became common among Africans and feared by Europeans. The institutionalization of official racial segregation, the creation of Pangani, the constant destruction of Africans' squatter settlements, and the allocation of the bulk of the city budget to improving services for the European community were all justified on medical grounds (that is, by the need to protect white settlers' health). Ironically, of course, such a system of urban "development" kept rates of infectious diseases high in the city, which in turn strengthened Europeans' arguments for segregation (53–54). As Obudho and Aduwo put it, after the first few years of settlement, "the political economy of health and disease tended to fossilize the incipient segregation" (54).

While Nairobi was being organized by notions of racial difference and disease, the colony as a whole was becoming segregated by gender. British officials defined the colonial city in all of its territories in sub-Saharan Africa as men's space; women's place was in the field. By 1920, the municipal government had in place a rigid pass-law system that regulated the entrance of Africans, especially women, to the city; a vagrancy law that allowed officials to arrest any African suspected of being unemployed; a housing "system" that provided no family-sized dwellings for Africans; and an economic structure that offered no opportunities for African women to earn a wage and, therefore, to avoid being targets of anti-vagrant campaigns (Cooper 1983, 7). The result was that Nairobi was an overwhelmingly male city; there were an estimated nine African men to every one African woman in the city before World War II (Kurtz 1988, 135).[2]

European officials had several reasons to keep African women out of the city. To maintain an economy based on low-wage migrant labor, it was enormously useful to have a labor force which could reproduce migrants at little or no cost to individual employers, the state, or capital in general. In most East African communities, much of the work of subsistence agriculture as well as of child-rearing and other components of reproduction was done by daughters and wives. Low male wages, whether paid in town, on white farms, or on construction projects, were subsidized by rural women.[3]

Another basis of the imperial interest in keeping women out of the city lay in colonial officers' dependence on the goodwill of rural chiefs. After removing many of them from the best agricultural land in the colony, most officials were anxious not to alienate rural patriarchs any more than was necessary. The elders of the villages and reserves from which most migrant workers came had a tacit agreement with the British; the elders would let their sons go to work for the white people but the British had to help keep the daughters and wives at home. If rural patriarchs lost control of young women's labor, sexuality, and progeny, then they lost their ability to use the promise of marriage and the importance of children and inheritance to pull young men back home (Stichter 1985). If rural patriarchs were to become too upset with the British, it would be hard for the latter to collect taxes or workers in the reserves. The system of "indirect rule" which the British applied to its African colonies depended on the willingness of rural patriarchs to serve as local agents of the imperial state. Without them, the state would be cut off from rural producers (Lewis 2000). Finally, all of these calculations were buttressed by the fundamental inability of most Europeans to imagine that African women had anything of value to offer them or their city.

Nevertheless, African women started moving to Nairobi as early as 1900, demonstrating their willingness to manipulate the colonial system to their own advantage. Luise White's fascinating and important history of the women who helped to settle Pumwani between the world wars demonstrates that women moved to colonial Nairobi for a variety of reasons. Some came to escape bad marriages and oppressive conditions on the reserves or in villages. Others came to earn cash to help their rural families survive economic crises. A few came to join their husbands after losing the family land or livestock to settlers or debts. Unable to get formal jobs, however, women migrants were often harassed and arrested for not having passes, vagrancy, illegal trading, or beer-brewing. Not infrequently, groups of young women who had come from the same part of the colony were rounded up and sent back to their villages (White 1990).

Much of the anxiety about women in the city was expressed in terms of the moral and medical dangers of prostitution. Urban Europeans' fears of syphilis were used to support arguments in favor of keeping women out of the city. Europeans, and many rural Africans as well, assumed that virtually every unmarried African woman in Nairobi was a prostitute. Of course, as White points out, the unequal ratio of men to women, the inability of many men to afford to bring a wife to the city, the absence of other cash-generating opportunities for women, the lack of social services for male workers, and a division of labor by gender that left single men in "need" of a woman to do their domestic work meant that selling sex, usually packaged with other "domestic" services, was a relatively common occupation among urban women. Pumwani's prostitutes provided urban African men with the same reproductive services as village and reserve women provided agricultural wage workers. Moreover, by doing this work cheaply, urban women subsidized the empire just as rural wives did.[4] According to officials and medical researchers alike, however, "prostitutes"—that is, all African women living in the city, however they were actually employed—were entirely responsible for the rising rates of syphilis in the African locations of Nairobi (Dawson 1983).[5] Unlike the supposedly temporary urbanization of male workers (a necessary evil), the urbanization of women apparently produced immorality, disease, and the breakup of the so-called traditional family, proving that female migration was dangerous and had to be contained.

By 1945, the ideological and material conditions that supported using racial and gender segregation as the solution to the real or imagined ills of Nairobi had been upset. As Nairobi struggled to absorb the large numbers of rural migrants and the nearly half-million Kenyan men returning from fighting in World War II, it became clear that evicting women and quarantining men could not solve the twin problems of prostitution and venereal disease, let alone any of the vast numbers of other more immediately deadly problems such as cholera and tuberculosis that were emerging in the city. New approaches to urban planning and urban policing were needed (Lewis 2000). They emerged in tandem with a reformulation of notions and representations of African bodies.

Historian Joanna Lewis (2000) argues that from at least the early twentieth century, two somewhat contradictory strands of racial-sexual thinking about Kenyans (and other peoples classified as "African") were evident. On the one hand was the well-entrenched belief that Africans were a less-evolved and therefore naturally and unchangeably beastly and depraved version of the species whose pinnacle of perfection had been achieved by the European.[6] This perspective had long been backed and elaborated by social and medical scientists determined to use Darwin's theory of evolution in the effort to classify the apparently very different peoples of the world. On the other hand was a perhaps gentler but unquestionably more paternalist and enduring view that Africans were like European children. As children they could be "raised" to maturity. Just how adult—that is, civilized or European-like—they could actually ever become was a matter of some disagreement. They could be raised "well" and become as happy and productive as their own characters and (questionable) abilities allowed. Or they could be raised badly, pushed to grow up too fast, given insufficient guidance, and allowed to run wild in a desperate, pathetic, and doomed imitation of their parents.[7] Should this latter scenario come to pass, "the white man" would have demonstrated that he had fumbled and dropped his famous burden of civilizing the nonwhite natives of the world.[8]

Joanna Lewis (2000) argues that the growing acceptance of the view among Europeans that Africans could be educated was closely linked to the efforts of many in the government to expand the colonial state; if the African was an educable child and if he was ever to run his own country properly, he[9] needed a benevolent parent-state big enough to ensure his proper training at every level. Not least among the relatively powerful champions of the reconstruction of the African character were the small but growing number of British medical doctors in the colony who were actually treating African patients. Lewis points out that until World War II, members of the colonial and missionary medical services were more intimately acquainted with the lives and troubles of individual Africans than were other Europeans, including those who used Africans as domestic servants. .

Arguments for African "uplift" were strengthened still further as demobilized African soldiers, anticipating at least some return from the empire on the investment they had made of their lives, came home. European settlers and officials alike began to fear that if disappointed, they might easily be persuaded to join the heretofore relatively fragmented and weak nationalist struggle.[10] Moreover, the war had flung black and white soldiers together and created new, more respectful and realistic, albeit still racist, views of Kenyan men among some Europeans (Lewis 2000). Lewis carefully documents the spurt of welfare provisioning that took place in the late 1940s and early 1950s in response to these changes. She notes that many demobilized soldiers were in fact successfully recruited by the colonial state as agents of state expansion in rural and urban areas.

Colonial civil servants in Nairobi took up the policy challenge offered by these changing conditions and perspectives. They argued that African "uplift" in the city required a concerted effort on the part of the state to mitigate the negative effects that too-rapid and too-sudden urbanization was having on the as-yet-immature African.[11] Medical and housing experts in particular urged the state to expand services for Africans in these two areas. According to Lewis, many of these experts believed that the solution to the apparent corruption of the urban African lay in doing just the opposite of what the government had been doing for so many years. Instead of discouraging women from migrating to the city, they insisted, the state should be encouraging "families"— that is, heterosexually married women and men—to settle permanently in the city (Lewis 2000). Prostitution and venereal diseases were inevitable in a city made up mostly of bachelors, they pointed out. The lack of houses or flats that were sufficiently large and sanitary for an African family and the lack of social and medical services for African women and children simply perpetuated the problem. Such experts urged the state to encourage women to come to the city and then provide them with the services and their husbands with the wages that would allow Africans to live in the working-class nuclear families that were idealized by the British and that would improve city life for all of Nairobi's residents.

The welfare officers were ultimately not very successful. Lewis argues that their attempts at state expansion and reform were thwarted by a combination of factors. Patronage relations between rural chiefs and government officials, shortages of resources available for African welfare, economic downturns in Britain, and, finally, violent white resistance followed by violent African resistance in the highlands blocked any real hope for long-term improvement in the living conditions of most Kenyans. One can see clearly the legacy of elitist neglect of working-class welfare in today's Nairobi.

The venereal-diseases clinic that was to become Casino, however, was one of the few "welfare" institutions the reformers did get built for Africans at this time. In the mid-1950s,[12] Casino opened its doors at the intersection of a still rigidly segregated urban space; the new health, economic, and political conditions and expectations of the postwar period; and the discovery that a single, cheap dose of penicillin could cure syphilis. The clinic's physical location left urban dwellers with no doubt that it was a clinic for Africans only. No such clinic was built for Europeans or for the Asians imported by the British to serve as an urban petit bourgeoisie; no members of either group were at all likely to find themselves seeking public medical treatment in the city's African location. The message was clear: only Africans get venereal disease and only Africans spread venereal disease.

Despite the racism expressed by its location, Casino provided a much-needed service. In 1944, officials reported that cases of syphilis among the Kikuyu, who made up the majority of Nairobi's African population, had increased by 20 percent since 1940.[13] Gonorrhea infections were also on the rise (Dawson 1988, 65). Much of this increase was the direct result not of urbanization but of the way that the sexual desires of soldiers of all nationalities posted around the empire were met by both official and unofficial prostitution during the war. It was the epidemic of syphilis among male soldiers in World War II that demonstrated that penicillin could be used inexpensively and on a massive scale to achieve astonishing results.[14]

In short, the concept and the building that I entered in March of 1993 had, like the idea and the shape of the city itself, been largely determined by the perceptions, interests, and needs of the colonial state. Colonial bureaucrats and settlers alike perceived African bodies as dangerous and diseased. The Colonial Office in London was interested in creating a "white man's" city to administer and support an economy for white settlers and the white metropole. To accomplish this, the Europeans needed to contain geographically, police, and reproduce cheaply the bodies of Africans who did most of the state's dirtiest work. They also had to provide a Band-Aid when their chosen system of reproduction resulted in potentially debilitating diseases and the threat of rebellion.

During the last years of British rule, state expansion and welfare provisioning in Nairobi came to a virtual halt. In 1952, Britain declared an official state of emergency; the government armed white settlers and increased restrictions on Africans' mobility in the face of the Mau Mau Rebellion (Robertson 1997). Urban Africans supported and joined the rebels in the forests around Nairobi and in the highlands. Feminist historians have demonstrated that Nairobi's prostitutes and women traders were among the first city-dwellers to join and energize the grassroots movement against the British. Their support incurred the wrath of the state, which landed on the official locations and the squatter settlements of Nairobi (Likimani 1985; Kershaw 1997; and Robertson 1997).

Mau Mau reinvigorated white racism. According to Maughan-Brown (1985), whites in Kenya unified and retrenched against organized African resistance. Once relatively liberal colonial officials joined conservative settlers and re-energized a racial ideology that represented the African as beastly and in need of violently delivered discipline. The colonial government returned briefly to the attempt to improve social services for Africans after British bombs put down the rebellion and the United States, now the world's greatest power, began worrying about the possible spread of communism in Africa. The racism of officials, combined with their awareness that the British empire was doomed (a reality that Kenya's settlers were not prepared to accept), kept their interventions minimal, however. Very little effort was spent on improving Nairobi; what work was done was devoted to rural community-building. Services for low-income urban residents were not expanded, despite the fact that rural poverty continued to motivate ever-increasing numbers of Kenyans to move to the city (Mburu 1992).

In the 1960s and early 1970s, Casino was affected by the new international discourses of development and modernization and by the institutions that were put in charge of these processes. In 1959, a technical officer specializing in venereal diseases arrived in Kenya from the World Health Organization's (WHO) headquarters in Geneva, Switzerland. His brief consultant's report (Lyall 1959) is the only description of Casino published before the clinic became a site for AIDS research in the late 1980s. In his report Lyall accomplishes two things. On the one hand, he reiterates and reinforces colonial notions about what he calls "African society's" fundamental difference from an assumed Europe. On the other hand, he at least partially translates the racially loaded discourse about "African" immorality into a vocabulary of "technical" observation and advice. I quote here the core of Lyall's report on "The Probable Extent of the Problem" of venereal disease in Kenya:

> While it would appear that African society does not shun the venereal disease patient, it was felt that attendance at the clinic might be encouraged by a change of title from "Venereal Diseases Clinic" to "Special Treatment and Skin Diseases Clinic." This recent change appears to have overcome the former reluctance of some known prostitutes to attend for treatment—a reluctance presumably due to fear of loss of custom [business] if it were known that the lady in question had contracted a venereal disease. (Lyall 1959, 2)

Lyall's words pay subtle homage to colonial notions about African sexual morality and how that morality demonstrates the enormous difference that exists between African and European. Lyall represents a homogenized "African society," perhaps approvingly, as tolerant of a problem, a type of patient, and an activity—heterosexual intercourse—about which British and American health officials were at this time very anxious and highly punitive (Brandt 1987). Simultaneously, Lyall approves of a renaming that he believes will erase the stigma associated with the old term "venereal." He confirms the importance of destigmatizing issues of sexual health by referring in a practical and morally neutral way to the needs of prostitutes.

Lyall's report continues in this apparently bipolar vein. He underscores the representation of African "difference" by providing—but neither explaining nor contextualizing—figures showing that "Africans" had rates of syphilis and gonorrhea infection that were, respectively, "26 times" and "33 times" the rates in English cities of equal size (Lyall 1959, 3). He does not mention that the relationship of Africans in Nairobi to Kenya is rather more analogous to the relationship of very poor Londoners to England than to the position of people in the British city of Preston that Lyall uses for comparison.

Lyall explicitly rejects the notion that venereal disease is caused by corruption and a "lack of family life" among Africans, however. He blames the high prevalence of syphilis and gonorrhea in the city on the poverty and limited employment opportunities produced for Africans, and particularly African women, by colonial development. This apparently destigmatizing translation, which characterized many such reports prepared for the WHO at this time, presages the emergence of the full-blown technocratic discourse on sexually transmitted diseases which the WHO produced from the 1960s on.[15]

In spite of Lyall's call for more attention to Casino and especially to the sexual health needs of Nairobi's women, the clinic was largely neglected by the government and the emerging international health development community in the years following Kenya's independence. During the 1960s, providing free quality health care to everyone was an important legitimizing strategy for the new state. Moreover, improving the health of Kenyans became a favorite object of development spending by the newly internationally conscious United States. Neither the urban working class nor sexual disease was considered important, however. Donors and the state spent virtually all monies for health care on building, staffing, and stocking maternal and child health care and family-planning clinics in the massively underdeveloped rural areas, training a desperately needed cadre of Kenyan doctors and nurses, and, much less appropriately, upgrading the already comparatively overdeveloped urban hospitals (Mburu 1992). Given this focus, it is hardly surprising that Kenya was wholly unprepared to meet the challenge of HIV/AIDS.

Casino continued to provide treatment to large numbers of patients every day, despite these considerable problems. It was the only free-standing venereal-diseases clinic in the entire country. Mombasa and Kisumu had small clinics inside their African-only hospitals, but these were used to treat professional prostitutes, often forcibly.[16] According to stories I heard from staff who had worked at the clinic for many years, lived in Nairobi all their lives, or heard stories from others, Casino was an overcrowded, understaffed, and highly stigmatized place through the 1960s, 1970s, and into the 1980s. Some of the older staff remembered one of the clinic's directors. They told me that this doctor had put his energy into making Casino's patients wish they had never come to the clinic. He would apparently yell at men and women whom he had treated once and who returned with a reinfection, sometimes refusing to treat them as punishment for their failure to keep "clean" or their failure to bring a sexual partner in for treatment. I was told that he assumed that all the women who came to Casino were prostitutes and that they were, therefore, beneath contempt.

By the time I arrived at Casino in 1993, decades of neglect combined with a series of economic crises had taken a visible toll on the clinic. One of the first things the clinic's head nurse said to me was that it was a very good thing for my clothes and notebooks that I had come in the dry season. "If you were here in the rainy season you wouldn't believe it. You would be all wet."[17] During the rains, patients waited for treatment in knee-deep water because the roof was all but gone. Because there was just one examination table in the clinic, only one person at a time could examine women. Casino's halls were always filled beyond capacity with waiting women squeezed tightly together on hard benches while trying to constrain restless small children. Men waited and were examined standing up. Bathrooms were broken and dirty. The clinic ran out of HIV- and even syphilis-testing kits with alarming frequency. It was a rare and much-celebrated occasion when Casino's lab had the equipment for doing diagnostic tests for anything other than blood-borne infections.

The possibility that HIV and other viruses were being spread within the clinic itself seemed quite strong, although no one was willing to discuss this possibility.[18] A single sterilization machine, which worked sporadically, had been serving the entire clinic for months. A nurse confided to me that they simply could not adequately sterilize the specula to keep up with the numbers of women waiting to be examined. Both women and men were often examined by staff who could not get gloves. The clinic did not have an adequate supply of disposable syringes or needles. There were no sealed containers to dispose of bloody needles or surplus blood samples. One staff member told me that some journalists had discovered used needles and syringes on the grounds around the clinic. The journalists tried unsuccessfully to get their story printed by the main daily paper. The staff member thought that the report should have been made public so the mayor or the president would do something to change the situation.[19]

In some respects, the arrival of HIV/AIDS had yet to change things materially at Casino, despite evidence that people at risk of contracting traditional STDs were typically at significant risk of being infected by HIV.[20] In fact, the discovery of the virus in the mid-1980s coincided with a deepening of Kenya's foreign-exchange crisis and the imposition of a structural adjustment program requiring the state to reduce spending on health care services. The supply of basic antibiotics had shrunk, and delivery was even more unpredictable than ever before. There were no drugs for HIV-related illnesses that were not sexually transmitted (such as cancer, pneumonia, thrush, or the massive loss of weight known as wasting). The sister-in-charge at Casino, Sister Njogo, summed up the drug situation on my first day at the clinic. She described the clinic's drug storeroom as "big and empty. It has nothing."[21]

Casino's colonial history continued to affect its current patients and its health care workers. One of the clinical officers informed me that young women fear they will be seen by family members or friends while they wait for the clinic to open; observers, he said, will assume the women are whores.[22] Although Casino's staff was often genuinely sympathetic with the patients, sometimes they revealed that they too were offended by the diseases that people, especially women, brought to the clinic.

On one particular day, the bench and hallways were exceptionally crowded. Word had spread in town that Casino had gotten a shipment of antibiotics and that patients would, therefore, be able to get their treatment at the subsidized state price instead of the much higher price charged at the nearby pharmacy. In her effort to keep some order in the hallway, Patricia spoke harshly to the waiting women. She told them that they were "*chafu,*" using the Kiswahili word for dirty, which, like the English word, can mean immoral as well as physically dirty. When I asked her later what she was telling the women, the nurse said in English: "They don't wash themselves at home. They know they are bad. They go to the toilet and don't wipe themselves so they are all full of stool. So if she knows she is bad she can wipe herself. But they don't wash."[23] None of the other staff milling around in the hallway that day commented on the nurse's phrasing. During my stay at Casino, such language came to seem almost normal. I never heard such language at the other clinics I visited. It seemed that to express disgust with the bodies of women with STDs was an accepted practice at Casino.

Nurses said that the stigma infected them as well. Ruth said that for years "everybody thought that the people who worked here had AIDS."[24] Wambui, who worked on the "female side," told me that she was trying to leave Casino. She wanted to get a job in a family-planning clinic and be free from the stigma and "dirt" of this notorious clinic. She was using her evenings, in fact, to undergo the extensive and difficult training required to become a family-planning nurse. The shortage of staff at Casino, however, made it unlikely that any of the nurses there would be allowed to leave.

In the early 1980s, just before the world discovered AIDS, Casino's luck began to change. A "global" site since its establishment by Kenya's foreign rulers, Casino's transnational identity started to be remade by a small group of Canadian STD doctors. In 1975 and 1977, there were two outbreaks of the sexually transmitted disease called chancroid[25] in the Canadian city of Winnipeg. According to STD researchers at the University of Manitoba in Winnipeg, prostitutes "appear[ed] to be the reservoir of disease" in these unusual outbreaks (Ronald and Albritton 1992, 263). In North America, chancroid is rare, and even in outbreaks it does not spread beyond very small populations. To learn more about the epidemiology and microbiology of chancroid, doctors Alan Ronald and Francis "Frank" Plummer went to Nairobi, where Kenyan researchers had already discovered that chancroid was very common. They got research permission from the national and municipal governments and the backing of the WHO's Collaborating Center on Sexually Transmitted Diseases, which Ronald had helped to establish a few years earlier.

From the perspective of the Canadian researchers, Casino was ideal. In order to test their theory about the relationship between prostitution and epidemic levels of chancroid among men, they needed a central location where it would be relatively easy to recruit a sufficiently large sample of female sex workers and their male clients at risk of getting chancroid. By 1983, Ronald and Plummer had set up shop in the rooms that the shortage of examination tables and drugs had left empty at Casino. From here they launched what would become probably the most important and influential medical research on the relationships between HIV and other STDs (Ronald, Plummer, and Ngugi 1991).

But it was not until the early 1990s, nearly ten years after these researchers had arrived, that health care workers at Casino started to see the material benefits of what had become in the interim a much larger, more internationalized, and better-funded project. The initial research project, and by extension Casino, suddenly became a focus of the international attention to health and sexuality in Africa that came in the wake of discoveries that African immigrants and white heterosexuals were getting HIV/AIDS. Many North American and Western European researchers and journalists had started to wonder aloud about whether their countries could learn something from the epidemic in sub-Saharan Africa that could help prevent the spread of HIV from small, apparently contained, "risk groups" to what was referred to as the "general public." Frank Plummer's group was prepared to answer this question.

By 1993, when I arrived at Casino, it was clear that HIV/AIDS research had affected daily life at Casino. On my initial tour of the clinic, Sister Njogo introduced me to what she and most of the staff called "the university side" of the clinic. The staff distinguished this side, in reality three square and windowless rooms off Casino's central corridor, from "the clinic side." The latter included the rooms off the "female hallway" on one side of the clinic, those off the "male hallway" on the opposite side, and several rooms along the back hallway where the laboratory, dispensary, injection, and "male" and "female" blood-drawing rooms were. When I asked about the researchers, several nurses said that they did not even know what "they are doing in those rooms" and that they believed it was none of their business to know.[26]

In practice, the line between university and clinic was blurry. The two sides shared the waiting rooms and bathrooms. Patients who met the criteria for whatever particular study or studies were going on at the time were always seen on the clinic side first. From there they were "referred," as the doctors and clinical officers put it, to the university side. Sometimes researchers would make use of the clinic's blood-testing equipment. Sister Njogo often visited the rooms on the university side to chat with the students or with the white research directors who occasionally stopped by. The university side was occupied mainly by Kenyan medical or nursing students working either for the Canadian STD team or the more recently established British team studying tuberculosis. The term "university" was appropriate for the Canadian team; they were based in two departments at the University of Nairobi's medical school. The British team, however, was not connected to an educational institution in Kenya at all, although they were loosely affiliated with the London School of Hygiene and Tropical Medicine. Nonetheless the staff put them all in the same category by virtue of their perceived purpose, their location within the clinic, and their foreign origins.

The university, or research, side was entirely dependent on the clinic—on the willingness and ability, that is, of the clinic's staff to send their patients to the researchers. Most of the patients diagnosed with HIV or AIDS[27] at the clinic were sent to one or another research project. When Sister Mithani, the nursing sister who was recruiting subjects for a study of HIV, was not getting a sufficient number of recruits, she had to change the criteria that the clinic staff would use to identify potential participants. She had been waiting for patients whose blood tested positive for HIV antibodies. The staff were sending too few patients to get tested, either because they had been told to use the tests sparingly or because they were too busy coping with the more evident STDs. The frustrated sister had to ask the staff to send her all the patients who had herpes zoster, a specific and visible sore; she expected that most of these patients would turn out to be HIV positive and therefore eligible for her study. Sister Mithani complained to me about having to teach the staff what the sore she was interested in looked like and said she had to monitor continually whether or not they were obeying her wishes.

The clinic side, in turn, was becoming ever more dependent on the university side. In the absence of the researchers and their foreign-funded and -directed AIDS projects, the terribly underresourced clinic could do next to nothing for HIV-positive patients. Apart from the research, Casino functioned as if the STD problem in Nairobi had never changed: syphilis and gonorrhea were the only diseases the clinic's staff could adequately address. Their ability to do even that was being severely curtailed by the drug shortage. They performed few blood tests for HIV; what was the point, the lab technician, Mr. Odhiambo, asked me, when they did not even have a regular HIV counselor on staff? Moreover, how could they decide who to test when the number of potentially infected patients was far greater than the supply of testing equipment? The university side offered what the clinic side could not give: testing, counseling, and comparatively good treatment and care. Clinic staff handed over suspected HIV/AIDS cases to the university side with relief and with the expectation, as I was told, that the transferred patients "were lucky; they would actually be cared for" if they were able to join the study. Once an HIV-positive patient had been referred to the university side, Casino's staff members were unlikely to see her or him again. This was another source of relief for the workers who were inadequately protected from being infected by their patients or by unclean instruments.

The researchers' presence promised to bring an even more direct benefit to the clinic. When I began my study at Casino, Sister Njogo and her staff were waiting for word on whether and when a project to renovate the clinic would materialize. A group of donor countries led by the European Union and Belgium had visited Casino not long before I arrived. Based primarily on research done first by the Canadian group and later by a Belgian woman studying at the University of London (Jenniskens 1992), the donors proposed to transform Casino into a referral clinic and laboratory for diagnosing and treating patients with HIV and more advanced STDs. This renovation and status change was to be done in conjunction with a Canadian project to train the staff of primary health care and maternal and child health care clinics to do "front-line" STD treatment. The idea was that all patients with STDs would first go to a primary health care clinic and that the nurses in these clinics would refer to Casino only those patients whom they could not treat.

Casino's staff had great expectations about how this project would improve the clinic and their working conditions. As she walked around Casino with me, Sister Njogo complained about the state of the clinic but also said, "We have a lot of hope. We are waiting for the people with deep pockets to fix these problems."[28] When I asked Mr. Mwalimu, a clinical officer trained by the Canadian team to work on the "clinic" side, how such a project might affect his work, he had no doubt that it would make all the difference for him. In my fieldnotes I paraphrased him: "He says it will make him feel like he is doing something. Now he writes prescriptions and the drugs are very expensive, even he can't afford them so these people [the patients] can't. He said, 'If there are drugs with the project, I will feel like I am doing something.'"[29]

When I left Casino three months later, however, Sister Njogo still did not know if or when the renovations would begin, despite the occasional visits that donor representatives and researchers had paid Casino during this period. She and her staff made it clear to me that all they could do was wait for the "deep pockets" of the foreigners; they had no faith that the municipal or national governments on their own would fix things at Casino. "It is up to our bosses, the EECs [European Economic Community], to do their task!" the sister said.[30]

The "globalization" of Casino lay not only in the presence of researchers or the promise of money from Europe and North America; it was visible in the materials of everyday work at the clinic. The HIV test kits that arrived sporadically were made in Great Britain and the United States. The specula came from Belgium. Some of the staff had been recently trained in STD management by the Canadian team of researchers. Other staff members were waiting for scholarships so that they could be trained in HIV counseling by the Swiss Red Cross. The boxes of condoms that sat on desks and tables in every room of the clinic were from the United States and were paid for mainly by the U.S. Agency for International Development (USAID). The antibiotics imported by the state or sometimes by the research projects came from multinational pharmaceutical companies headquartered in the United States and Great Britain. The white coats and dresses worn by the staff were often purchased from women selling bales of used American clothing. My presence there at that time is part of this globalization. I was at Casino thanks to the help of the Canadian research team, some members of which were interested in learning what a social scientist might discover. Several times Sister Njogo expressed the hope that I could help motivate the "deep pockets" by writing about the clinic's problems and needs.[31]

The cumulative effect of Casino's development since the mid-1980s was to make AIDS foreign. For the staff on the clinic side, AIDS as a concept or object of knowledge and action—as distinct from the presence of HIV revealed by the antibody tests—existed behind the closed doors and in the off-site laboratories of the foreign-funded researchers. It existed as a reason why foreign countries were promising to upgrade the clinic. It was not really present in the everyday negotiations between clinic staff and patients or among the staff. None of the staff—nurses, doctors, clinical officers, cleaners—was very interested in talking about AIDS. For the most part, they had no idea who was HIV positive and who was not. When I asked them why, they shrugged or said they did not think such knowledge was really relevant to their work.

The staff members' apparent disinterest in AIDS, evident at a time when the national government was beginning to be more open about the crisis, surprised me. The nurses were neither ignorant nor in denial about HIV's existence or significance. They did not express what continued to be a popular view among Kenyans, that HIV had been produced in American labs in order to reduce the size of Africa's population. I came to believe that what seemed like disinterest was more likely an awareness that to address AIDS in a serious way would require supplies of money that could only come from outside the country. Given the shortages at Casino, the ability of the staff to do anything for HIV-infected patients or for their patients who were at risk of getting HIV (virtually all of Casino's patients) was limited to treating their other STDs or sending them off to join a research project. What capacity Nairobi's public clinics had at the time, or could have in the future, resulted exclusively from foreign funds and the interests that determined how those funds would be spent.

While they generally pushed AIDS out of the main clinic and into the rooms of the university side, thereby limiting the extent to which AIDS directly influenced their everyday work, staff members did use notions about sexual risk associated with HIV/AIDS as well as other STDs to organize, diagnose, and advise their patients. A central argument of this book is that what Nairobi's public health nurses told me about their patients' sexuality reflected the nurses' positions as *brokers* of exchanges taking place in the clinic between local patients and transnational researchers, clinic needs and foreign "pockets," and colonial agendas and development policies.

Although the stories that Casino's nurses told me about their patients and the translations they offered me of their interactions with patients varied and sometimes contradicted each other, they grew from several shared assumptions. They were always premised on a belief that everyone (including the staff members and me, the audience) was heterosexual. During my fieldwork there, no one at Casino referred in any way to the possibility of same-sex sexual transmission, despite the fact that the clinic's staff routinely treated prisoners from Nairobi's prison for men.[32] In addition, staff members appeared to agree that a patient's ethnic, tribal, or religious affiliation was relevant to their sexual behaviors, relative risk of infection, or sexual identities.[33] A patient's socioeconomic class position was rarely directly spoken about. In general, Casino was, and is, perceived to be a clinic for the poorer people in Kenya's working class, including those generating small incomes as self-employed hawkers, handymen, domestic workers, or prostitutes. So STDs were already defined for the health care workers as a class-specific problem, as a problem of the poor. No one challenged this except to note, occasionally, that the city's very poorest people were not likely to show up at the clinic because they could not afford the bus ride, let alone the cost of drugs.

The most important and explicit of the shared assumptions was that gender is the most important factor determining the nature of patients' risk. Casino's staff, however, defined feminine gender and masculine gender as forces operating in quite different ways. Not only do women and men experience the effects of being gendered individuals quite differently and unequally, but gender itself is qualitatively different for men and women. According to workers at Casino, femininity is not a property possessed or performed by an individual. For women patients, gender is a set of sexual, economic, and health-related relationships between biological males, females, and children. At least in the context of their work at Casino,[34] staff members agreed that the risk faced by Casino's female patients is determined by how their marital status ties them sexually and reproductively to men as husbands, boyfriends, or clients. In contrast, masculine gender, defined primarily in terms of sexual behavior, is a property of the individual male body (or at least of what the nurses usually called the "African" male body). Although some masculine behaviors may be influenced by the nature of a man's relationship to a given woman, masculine sexuality, the core of masculine identity, is an essentially constant, unvarying and individual performance.

The consensus that gender gave men and women fundamentally different experiences and needs with respect to STDs was evident from the moment I entered Casino's courtyard. Before the clinic's doors opened in the morning, guards organized the patients waiting outside into two lines, men on the left and women (with or without children) on the right. Women and men entered separate waiting areas and were registered by different clerks. Men were then directed into the "male hallway," where they were seen by one of the three male clinical officers who worked exclusively on the male side. The much larger group of women and children filed into the "female hallway" to wait for their turn to be examined by the clinic's one medical doctor, a male gynecologist with a rudimentary understanding of STDs in women and no interest in treating men.

According to nurses, this sex segregation reflected more than the material reality of having only one room with an examination table. They did not expect that an increase in the number of such tables would end the segregation because, as Wambui put it, she "would feel uncomfortable" if men and women mixed at the clinic, and, she thought, women patients would also be "uncomfortable."[35] Moreover, the "healthy talk" that patients of both genders were supposed to get from nurses every day differed depending on the gender of the audience. In fact, during my three-month stay, men never got a "healthy talk." Women, on the other hand, received talks relatively regularly.

The explicit segregation and the implicit policy of targeting only women with education about STD treatment and prevention were consistent with an almost-overwhelming consensus among the staff about masculine heterosexuality. Health care workers, male and female, agreed that whether by nature or by tradition Kenyan men were sexually irresponsible and untrustworthy. Dr. Gitau, a Kenyan male clinical officer,[36] told me quite simply that men "are irresponsible; it's difficult to deal with them."[37] Sister Njogo summed up a view I found to be common among the nurses when she said with disgust, "You can't trust men [to use a condom]. Condoms don't work because the men are drunk so they tear the condoms to get skin to skin."[38] The view that men always want "skin to skin" when they have vaginal intercourse with a woman was repeated by a number of nurses. One nurse added that "he tears it to prove that it is so weak, that they [condoms] do bust." The sister explained further that many men would not use condoms because they still held a "traditional belief that if a man has [an STD or HIV], having a negative wife will be medicine." Her disapproval of this belief was clear; she pointed out that "of course, what really happens is that now she [the HIV-negative woman] is infected too."[39]

Men's irresponsibility was not limited to their unwillingness to use condoms. Men's apparent tendency to resist pressures to bring their sexual contacts in for treatment was also frustrating to the staff. Dr. Oludho, another male clinical officer, was troubled because he could not get men to bring in their female sexual partners to get treated. "It is very difficult to get men to bring their contacts. I tell them to bring them but there is nothing I can do. They might tell you 'She is very far out of Nairobi.' To convince them it is for their own good is very difficult."[40] Ruth repeated this account almost verbatim when she warned me, "If you are not careful, they will not tell you they got [the STD] in Nairobi. They'll say they got it from far away, Mombasa, Kisumu. They will even tell you their wife is far away."[41]

There were other frustrations with men. Mr. Mwalimu gave me a more humorous but still telling example of men's irresponsibility. He reported that on Fridays, if word is out in the community that Casino has drugs, men will come in and ask for a drug that will give them "protection" when they have sex over the weekend. The clinical officer said that he tells the men: "Okay, I can give you something but there are many different things you can catch. You can catch gonorrhea, you can catch syphilis, you can catch AIDS. So if you tell me which one you are going to catch, I can give you something!"[42] Saying this, he laughed and threw his hands up in the air in a gesture of helplessness. With much less humor, Sara told me that men were less likely to come to Casino for treatment than women: "Men have already gone to private doctors. . . . As soon as a man is sick he goes off to private; he only comes here with complications. They come here and cause problems" because, as she explained, private doctors trying to make a profit will frequently give their patients an inadequate dose of antibiotics; when the infection returns, now resistant to the original drug, the man will finally show up at Casino.[43]

The nurses threw men's irresponsibility into even greater relief by comparing their "African" masculine behavior to that of "European" (white) men. After complaining about "men's" irresponsibility, they would assure me that "*Wazungu*" men were not as bad as "African" men. I could not get the nurses to tell me whether they said this because they were worried about my sexual future, because they thought I believed this and wanted to hear them say it, or because they really believed it. It was a fairly common refrain, in any case. Several times I was asked, only partly in jest, "Karen, when you go home, bring me back an *Mzungu* to marry—along with a new nurse's uniform!" Such binary constructions of irresponsible African men versus sexually controlled European men reverberate with colonial ideas and representations of savage and sexually dangerous black men. But in focusing on masculinity's role in STD and HIV prevention, the nurses challenged researchers' and development experts' obsession with transmitting women, a problematic to which I will return later.

In short, the staff had little sympathy for men who had STDs. Male clinical officers and female nurses alike expressed frustration, disgust, anger, and occasionally cynical humor about men's "irresponsibility" toward sex and health. They also seemed to expect and even count on such irresponsibility; their stories indicated their resignation and a view that men's behavior was traditional, predictable, and inevitable. The tacit agreement not to give men "healthy talks" reflected the staff's expectations about masculinity. If men qua men are irredeemably irresponsible, what would be the point in wasting precious and limited staff time trying to educate them?

The staff told very different stories about women. Ruth described women as "good patients who are less complicated than men."[44] "Complicated" here, it seems, translates as "irresponsible." Women were also expected to care about their children's health. I frequently heard the gynecologist tell his patients that they needed to take care of their STDs, if not for themselves then for the babies they might have in the future.

The "healthy talks" that I listened to while waiting in the crowded female hallway revealed some of the contrasts between views of femininity and masculinity. In my fieldnotes, I paraphrased in English a typical "healthy talk" for women, delivered in Kiswahili:

> It starts with an introduction to what is an STD. [The nurse says,] "It is a disease caused especially by adulterous or immoral sex [*magonjwa ya zinaa*].[45] Women will have a discharge. Gonorrhea can also cause blindness in babies if a woman who has it gives birth. Another is syphilis."
>
> Then J. [the nurse] pulls out a condom and stretches it between her two hands while she continues to talk. "We will take blood and test it to see if this is syphilis. If you are spotted or have marks [*madoadoa*] on your face, go to the doctor instead of just staying at home. This is herpes.
>
> "To avoid getting these diseases have one friend [*rafiki;* here, boyfriend or sexual partner]. Two or three is dangerous and you will get AIDS [*ukimwi*]. Don't be a prostitute [*malaya*]. Use a condom to avoid *magonjwa ya zinaa*. The man wears the condom to avoid passing an infection. If you agree with each other, you can use the male condom. After using it once, throw it into the toilet; it's bad if the children get it. Dispose of it well and do not use it more than once. For women there is a need for a female condom, but there is not one yet. Any questions?"
>
> One woman asks a question about when to use a condom.
>
> J. says you can't use a condom unless you agree with each other. "Listen and talk to each other [*sikilizana*]. The condom is to avoid both STD [said in English] and pregnancy."
>
> After a few more questions, J. mimes washing her body, squatting and rubbing her arms and breasts. R., another nurse, talks about hygiene [*hygieni*] being a good thing. "Wash like this [points to J.] morning and evening. Wash under your arms and breasts. This is the lesson about hygiene. Any questions?"
>
> R. then walks around the hallway holding out to the women an open box of wrapped condoms. Some women take a few, most take none. J. keeps talking about how it is necessary that the women go to the doctor, "otherwise you could die. Don't go to the chief or the traditional healer [*daktari wa zamani*]. Go to the hospital and you can get better."[46]

This talk raised a number of important issues about women's experiences and needs. For our purposes here, the most important message of the talk was that some of the women in the audience, unlike any of the men waiting on the other side of the clinic, could be expected to do something to prevent STDs. The nurses repeatedly told women, as a group and, in certain cases, individually, that they could choose to have only one partner or "friend." Women were expected to try to negotiate with their partner and even convince him to use a condom. They should be able to identify their own diseases and could prevent them from getting worse by inspecting and washing their bodies and avoiding traditional medicine.

While we sat in the examination and treatment rooms where the nurses counseled women patients who had been diagnosed as having an STD and maybe HIV, the nurses categorized their women patients based on the logic that femininity and feminine "risk" are relational phenomena. According to the nurses, the kind of counseling or advice a woman needed depended not so much on her own sexual or economic behavior but on how the nature of her relationship to a man or to men as a group could be expected to determine his or their sexual, economic, and health-seeking behavior.

Most of the nurses premised their advice to women patients on the view that women's risk could vary depending on the kind of health-seeking behavior the men with whom she was sexual could be expected to exhibit. When talking to me about men, the nurses represented African masculinity as homogenously irresponsible. When they were discussing heterosexual relationships with women patients, however, the nurses identified different masculine behaviors that had crucial meaning for women's risk of sexual disease. There were three categories of heterosexual men: the *bwana* (husband), the *rafiki* (boyfriend), and the *marafiki* (multiple boyfriends and/or clients).

Bwana can be expected (by their wives and by nurses as they talk to wives) to come in for treatment. The nurses put a lot of pressure on women with *bwana* to inform them of the infection and to bring them to Casino for treatment. "We told her not to come back without her *bwana;* maybe we won't treat her if she fails to bring him," Celeste told me as she translated her conversation with a Kikuyu woman infected with syphilis.[47] The nurses asserted that as a husband, a man can be convinced to come in for treatment. Because he is married to the infected woman and because it is likely that he does or will share children with her, he is the most likely of men to want and accept treatment.

There is a limit to a *bwana*'s responsibility for his wife's health, however. Nurses almost never gave condoms to women with *bwana*. Rarely did they even suggest condom use to these women. I asked about this on most occasions because I knew that the nurses were supposed to insist that every single patient take condoms. The nurses who did not just shrug at my obviously ridiculous question told me that as a *bwana* a man "would never use a condom." "A wife would be beaten for suggesting such a thing" because by doing so she is implying that either she or the *bwana* had been "going out" (sleeping around). Quite simply, it was very dangerous to the immediate survival of a wife for a nurse to advise her to try condoms, even if as a man he cannot be expected to change his "irresponsible" sexual behavior.

Unlike women with *bwana,* women with *rafiki* are not expected or exhorted to bring their partners in (despite the wishes and expectations of researchers). "But if [her partner] is a *rafiki* [friend or lover], we have to consider. He can be a partner for one day and no way a patient can get [him to come]; but if it is a husband . . . we advise them [women patients] that a good *bwana* will come."[48] Without sexual and reproductive claims legitimized by marriage, female partners of male *rafiki* have no power over masculine "irresponsibility," say the nurses.

Women with *rafiki* are pressed to take condoms, however. They are also frequently encouraged to "*acha rafiki*" (roughly translated as "dump the guy"). Women with irresponsible *rafiki* can and should see themselves as capable of being on their own, without a man (I never heard a nurse suggest to an unmarried woman that she get married). Women with *bwana,* however, are never told to leave their husband, however irresponsible or even violent he may get. So, according to the nurses, women with *rafiki* have, or should have, a different kind of sexual agency from that of women with *bwana.*

Women with "*marafiki*" ("many" boyfriends, probably more than three or four) might be sex workers. As such, they clearly do not deserve much respect or gentleness from the nurses—as the often-hostile and even yelled "counseling" conversations with such women suggested to me. But several of the nurses I observed and interviewed chose not to assume that a woman with multiple boyfriends should be defined as a prostitute. They did not assume that such women, regardless of their income sources, were responsible for their infections. Even the more hostile nurses registered the (epidemiologically correct but frequently ignored) view that whether or not a woman took money for having sex with several different men was irrelevant to her risk of infection. Moreover, they frequently expressed an opinion similar to that of one nurse, who told me that having multiple sexual partners probably would not stop as long as women are poor. Ruth put it in pragmatic terms: "It's not easy to tell her to stop the business. What else is she going to do? Sell tomatoes? [I tell her] 'Try to get another type of business [but] if you have to continue being a prostitute, you have to use condoms as far as possible.'"[49] Sister Njogo was equally nonjudgmental. She blamed irresponsible men for turning women and girls into prostitutes. Men, she said, "are really the prostitutes. They bring women around and the women have no place to go. . . . On Koinange Street, those cars that drive by pick [up] the girls and the girls have nowhere to go."[50] The matron and the nurses repeatedly referred to men's irresponsibility and drunkenness, not women's morality, as the biggest threats to women who sell sexual services.

The perception that women were educable with regard to protecting themselves and their children from STDs, albeit along different dimensions determined by their marital and sexual situation, was linked with the presumption that unmarried women could reduce the number of sexual partners they had. The linking of these two views of women led nurses and clinical officers to conclude that women, unlike men, were not only sexually more responsible in a positive sense but that women could be held responsible for, that is, blamed for, not preventing STDs.

Health care workers' constructions of African masculine sexual behavior as the result of moral and biological irresponsibility and their opposing but more complicated representation of women as good patients and culpable sexual agents express the central contradiction that is the empirical focus of this book. According to health care workers, medical researchers, and policymakers, men contribute enormously to the spread of HIV in Kenya by being sexually, reproductively, economically, and socially irresponsible but women are and should be the main targets of local, national, and international attempts to stop the epidemic.

Although there have been many changes at Casino during the more than thirty years since Kenya's independence, there is significant continuity in the discourse about heterosexuality and responsibility. The view that African men who left their villages for the big cities, mines, or soldier camps of the colonized subcontinent were sexually and morally irresponsible was a constant refrain in the health and welfare policies of the colonial government as well as of much of the medical science being produced contemporaneously (Dawson 1983; White 1990; Curtin 1998; Lewis 2000). By the 1940s, colonial representations of urban African women in Nairobi were shot through with contradictions similar to some of those underlying practices at Casino in the 1990s. As we have seen, the migration of single women to the city was viewed as a dangerous threat to the health of African men and, by extension, to the European community. Prostitutes and women living with their urbanized husbands, however, provided the infrastructure for a more stable, potentially less-demanding population of low-paid wage-earning men (White 1990; Lewis 2000). African women have long been viewed by colonial and independent states as well as by development experts as simultaneously more trustworthy, stable, and teachable than men and as more culpable than men for problems as wide-ranging as overpopulation, high infant mortality, environmental degradation, loss of food self-sufficiency, and HIV/AIDS (Hartmann 1995). These external and internal, historical and contemporary, local and global forces give form and content to health care workers' negotiations with and stories about their patients.

Three

Negotiating AIDS
Policy in Kenya
1984–1994

Over the last twenty years, Kenya's official and unofficial responses to HIV/AIDS have been shaped by what Cindy Patton calls the "invention of African AIDS" (1990). This process took place largely, but not entirely, outside of sub-Saharan Africa, orchestrated mainly by medical and social scientists, journalists and editors, politicians and bureaucrats in the United States, Britain, France, and Switzerland. It is an invented discourse that, among other things, obliterated the role of past and present social, political, and economic inequality between nations, races, classes, sexualities, and genders in creating the current crisis.

According to Cindy Patton, the "African paradigm" was based on three claims or assumptions. One was that one could speak of "Africa" as a single entity despite the fact that there is greater social, political, linguistic, and cultural diversity on the continent than in North America and Western Europe combined. Moreover, the idea that Africa was synonymous with AIDS trumped emerging evidence that infection levels varied considerably by region, among cities, and in different groups of people. Some scientists also knew, but could not get the word out, that there were large parts of the continent (mainly the western and northern areas) that had few or no cases.

A second premise of the paradigm was that Africans were unable to diagnose AIDS correctly. This belief led North American and European researchers to reject the arguments of many Central and Eastern African physicians that their patients with AIDS did not look different from their patients without AIDS; those with AIDS got the same infections that were already common in the communities where they lived

47

(Chirimuuta and Chirimuuta 1989). African physicians' warnings that diagnostic criteria developed in Europe and the United States were unsuitable for their patients were typically dismissed. According to Richard and Roseline Chirimuuta, some African doctors found that the first test kits used to identify HIV antibodies could not distinguish HIV from malarial infection. Claims that there were extremely high numbers of Africans already infected in the early 1980s were incorrect. Although North American and European researchers eventually caught on to the problem, for years they simply accepted the inflated statistics as proof that the virus originated in Africa.

The third premise of the paradigm, according to Patton, was derived from colonial constructions of "darkest" Africa as the source of evil, usually taking the form of terrible diseases. Several scholars have pointed out just how readily such constructions were revived in the attempt to explain heterosexual AIDS (Gilman 1988; Sabatier 1988; Watney 1989a and 1989b; Treichler 1999). AIDS had to be a natural condition of Africa because Africans are by nature sexually promiscuous (even perverted), went the argument. They are also naturally poor and backward; the apparent absence of capitalist industrialization on the continent completed the explanation for why AIDS was spreading among African heterosexuals (and, by implication, why it probably would not spread among white heterosexuals living in the apparently successfully industrialized countries of the world).[1]

Why now, nearly twenty years later, do we need to remember this early construction of heterosexual AIDS as a puzzle that scientists and journalists Africanized into something both understandable to and safely far away from their Euro-American audiences? Susan Sontag (1989) has argued that we frequently create simplistic and accusatory systems to explain a new disease. She asserts that when biomedical knowledge finally catches up and gives us the truth, we eventually drop these systems. Medical researchers have very quickly learned much about HIV and the reasons it spreads more rapidly and widely in some populations than in others. Hundreds, perhaps thousands, of articles based on good scientific research in many countries of Africa have been published; researchers have demonstrated the complexities of HIV on the continent. Those early racist notions are certainly regrettable, but we have now moved on, no?

In some respects, North American and European social scientists, medical researchers, and journalists have become more sophisticated and more sensitive in our analyses. It is somewhat unusual today to find stories about "AIDS in Africa" that do not make clear which countries and cities are actually being talked about, for example. A relatively new solidarity among AIDS activists in the United States, Europe, and especially Southern Africa has emerged out of crucial conversations concerning the availability, cost, and side effects of treatments; the power of pharmaceutical companies; the politics of trade agreements; and the ethics of clinical trials. This solidarity is premised on a much more complicated understanding of what people with HIV in different parts of the world have in common and also how the conditions of their lives differ.

The "African AIDS" paradigm remains embedded in how we continue to think about AIDS and about Africa, however. When I tell people that I am writing about the politics of AIDS in Kenya, many of them gasp and say something such as, "Isn't it horrible? The continent is being wiped out, right? What a depressing subject." Of course AIDS is horrible. It is a horrible set of diseases, a horrible thing to live with, and a horrible way to die. The comments I get, however, carry astonishing generalizations about "the continent" and the "devastation." My audiences unwittingly imply that the "horror" is still particularly African; it does not seem to exist here in the United States or anywhere else in the world (in spite of very good data to the contrary). Moreover, today it seems that Africa and AIDS are virtually synonymous in the U.S. media. In June of 2002, I picked up a local paper in Durham, North Carolina. A respected AIDS researcher had written the cover story, which was headlined: "AIDS Is Not a Gay Disease. African Diary: A UNC-Chapel Hill Researcher's Odyssey through the Beauty and Devastation of an AIDS-Plagued Continent" (Van der Horst 2002).[2] Are we to believe from this title that, like its beauty, Africa's AIDS plague is natural, part of the scenery? Must we choose whether AIDS is a gay (apparently not African) or an African (apparently not gay) disease? Are we still to understand Africa as a single place and Africans as a single category of persons with respect to HIV/AIDS?

The "African paradigm" is still apparent in more academic publications as well, albeit in forms that are somewhat reorganized and usually subtler than those that appeared in the past. For example, the 2001 edition of an important college textbook on African political and social issues includes a five-page section on AIDS (Gordon 2001). The editors of this textbook, one of whom authored this section, have amply demonstrated elsewhere their sophisticated and in-depth knowledge of the enormous variety of historical experiences and social, cultural, and political organizations on the continent. But in this section these differences disappear, collapsed into that same single entity "African AIDS." Here again, the paradigm is invoked; AIDS is exclusively heterosexual, associated with prostitution (the nature of which we are assumed to know) and male sexual infidelity. It is caused by "poverty." Virtually all African governments continue to deny its existence.[3] African AIDS is a result of distinctly African problems; internal variations are trivialized and no reference is made to the influence of past or present global economic relations. The author perceives the "international" as simply a necessary source of "pressure" on and financial assistance to African states.

How and why has this paradigm persisted in the face of so much evidence against it? One reason is that there has been little attempt by the producers of popular culture in the United States to educate its citizens about AIDS or anything else in Africa. More important for AIDS experts, however, is that very early in the epidemic, the paradigm was enshrined in an apparently scientific schema that the WHO put forward and widely circulated in specialist and popular scientific media alike. In their widely cited 1988 article, Peter Piot, now the head of the Joint UN Programme on HIV/AIDS (UNAIDS); Jonathan Mann, the first director of the WHO's Global Programme on AIDS (GPA); and Frank Plummer, the director of the AIDS/STD project in Nairobi asserted that in contrast to the United States and Western Europe, AIDS in Africa is about sexual behavior (promiscuity), not sexual orientation (homosexuality):

> The initial assessments of the AIDS epidemic in African countries revealed a very different epidemiology from that in Western countries. Level of sexual activity with multiple partners, not sexual orientation, was the apparent risk factor. . . . Over the past 2 years, evidence has emerged that partially elucidates the mechanisms of this dichotomy. (Piot et al. 1988, 574)

The rather startling comment that "sexual orientation" is relevant—indeed a risk—in the "Western countries"[4] but not in Africa and that having multiple partners is relevant in Africa but not in Europe or the United States implies both that heterosexuality is not a sexual orientation and that it is being homosexually oriented, not sexually active, that puts (all) people of the "West" (but not Africans) at risk. This construction was not consistent with what many scientists and activists already knew about HIV by the time this article was published. "Orientation" does not transmit the virus, and spread of the virus by unprotected sexual activity is not fundamentally different among different groups of people (Farmer 1992). Nevertheless, the perception that there are two different "AIDS," one caused by behaviors that are perhaps racially and/or geographically specific and the other caused by orientation, lies at the heart of the schema that the WHO developed between 1986 and

1988 and that continues to organize international scientific and development thinking about the crisis.

The WHO's description of the global epidemiology of HIV was based on the "discovery" that there were two different "patterns" of infection and that these patterns seemed to be linked to specific geographic regions. "Pattern one" (Western Europe and the United States are always first) was characterized by high rates of infection among "homosexuals" and some spread among intravenous drug users and hemophiliacs but very low rates of infection among heterosexual women.[5] In the Latin American, Caribbean, and sub-Saharan African countries that followed "pattern two," by contrast, heterosexual women seemed as likely to be infected (or to have AIDS) as men. Perinatal transmission was common in these countries as well. These facts indicated that heterosexual sex constituted the main way in which HIV spread in "pattern two" countries. "Pattern three" countries were countries that seemed to have very few cases; that is, North African, Middle Eastern, and Asian countries. Later, however, these countries were described as demonstrating a combination of the first two patterns of spread.[6]

The construction of epidemiological patterns—that is, the reframing of "difference" in apparently scientific, objective, and politically neutral terms—probably helped to defuse the hostilities that emerged in the mid-1980s over who was to blame for the disease. Between 1984 and 1986, a series of accusations and counteraccusations was lobbed across the Indian and Atlantic Oceans. Western European and U.S. researchers hypothesized that the newly identified virus causing AIDS had come to their countries from Central Africa via Haiti (Farmer 1992). Some Haitian, Zairian, and Kenyan journalists and politicians argued that the virus must have originated in the "West" since it was obviously a "gay" disease and homosexuality was a "Western" perversion. An early symposium on AIDS held in Brussels ended in a standoff between a group of European and North American medical scientists who claimed that AIDS originated in Africa and was spreading fast all over the subcontinent and Africans who said that the Euro-American obsession with African origins made doing something about the disease more difficult (Chirimuuta and Chirimuuta 1989, 122). The fifty African representatives at the symposium issued a statement asserting their position that there was no evidence proving that AIDS came from Africa (122–123).[7]

Nonetheless, tensions continued to grow. In 1986, several European and Asian countries launched racist offensives to "protect" their citizens from AIDS by expelling or threatening to expel African students and visitors. For their part, several African governments refused to admit that there were significant numbers of AIDS cases in their countries.

This denial, in which Kenya's President Moi enthusiastically participated, was due at least in part to an understandable fear that their
countries would lose essential tourist dollars. Reports that British and
American travel agents were cautioning their clients about tainted "African" blood supported the government's fears. President Moi claimed
that the furor over AIDS was just another attempt by the United States
and Europe to blame Africa for things that were really the result of our
own immorality (Sabatier 1988).

In this context, the WHO's attempt to reframe "difference"—and to
do so without the slightest reference to origins—was no doubt welcome.
It seemed nonjudgmental and neutral; in it, no country or individual
is bad or deviant, perverted or backward. Countries are simply "pat-
terned." At the same time, however, the pattern model reimposed in
new forms an old notion of fixed sexual difference tied to geographical
and racial boundaries. This representation of difference, however scientifically rephrased, clearly misrepresented the shape and dynamism of
the epidemic as it spread to virtually all parts of the world. The representation continued to influence both research and policy in Kenya well
into the 1990s.[8]

During the 1950s and early 1960s, politicians and scholars embraced
the notion that the newly independent countries of Africa and Asia could
"catch up" to their former colonial rulers by adopting the institutions, technologies, sciences, and attitudes that those rulers had produced. A crucial aspect of the new emphasis on development as "modernization" and "westernization" involved the diffusion of biomedical
thinking, technology, and practices directly to Africans in the class-
rooms of brand-new foreign-funded medical schools; in packages of imported drugs, contraceptives, immunizations, and blood-test kits; and
through research trips by British and North American biomedical experts. By the time Kenya gained its independence in 1962, the WHO
was the champion and manager of this transnational flow.

Although the WHO had encountered a number of international health
crises before, AIDS presented at least two new challenges. One was the
challenge AIDS made to the knowledge and perspectives of international health experts. The other challenge was to the very identity of the
organization. Until the mid-1980s, international health experts basi-
cally believed that fatal infectious diseases had been entirely defeated in
the so-called industrialized countries and that, thanks to biomedicine,
the rest of the world was on an irreversible, albeit slow, path away from
infectious diseases toward lower mortality, longer life expectancy, and
fewer so-called lifestyle diseases such as lung cancer, heart disease,
and diabetes (Kunitz 1987). AIDS came as a shock to a great many

people in the field of health and development; experts were simply unprepared both ideologically and intellectually. The sexually transmitted disease program, which was very important under the brief tenure of the League of Nations' health organization, had been all but shut down by the time AIDS came along. Immunology was a marginal field even in the wealthy countries; virtually no one at the WHO had any knowledge of this area.

Moreover, the WHO found itself at the center of a set of struggles over the definitions of AIDS, risk, sexuality, and sexual deviance, that is, over the politics of health and death. This proved to be problematic for an organization that had long prided itself on making recommendations that were politically neutral, noninterventionist, and scientifically sound. Indeed, it was this supposed neutrality that led the WHO to dub itself the organization most capable of leading the world's governments out of the apparent chaos of half-truths; racist, nationalist, and homophobic accusations and discrimination; and widespread fear and uncertainty.[9] An official history of the early years of the WHO's AIDS program makes explicit this view of the WHO's role as both necessary and difficult:

> WHO's policy and strategy development through 1985–7 was seen both inside and outside the organization as an attempt to create order out of chaos. . . . Although it did not initiate every event, GPA was expected to take part, and often to lead. The uncertainties were political and ethical as well as epidemiological. . . . Although WHO had earned respect for a number of its other programmes, never before had it been in the position of counsellor, arbiter, and opinion-leader over such a sensitive and high-profile issue. (WHO 1992a, 5)

It was its self-presentation as politically neutral and the widespread acceptance of that representation that made it the ideal leader of the global battle to come. But the WHO's director-general, Halfdan Mahler, soon realized that in order to confront the highly politicized chaos, the WHO would have to risk that same reputation of neutrality, develop a clear stand on how governments should perceive AIDS and cope with it, and be explicitly interventionist to ensure that governments complied.

The WHO did not respond immediately when the first cases of the new and apparently spreading syndrome were identified in 1981 (Gellman 2000). In fact, a number of communities first affected by the disease and, more disastrously, by AIDS-related discrimination—white gay men in the United States, sex workers in the United States and

Europe, Haitian immigrants in the United States, and Central African immigrants to Western Europe—accused the WHO of being as indifferent to them as their own governments. Mahler finally called a few experts together in Atlanta in 1983. Even at this point, two years into what many were already realizing might be a very serious international crisis, the WHO resisted pressures to take a leading role. Mahler did make an important, albeit indirect, statement against racism, however, when he concluded publicly that there was insufficient evidence to support American, French, and British claims that AIDS originated in Africa (WHO 1984).

In 1986, fully three years after the Atlanta meeting and two years after the virus then called HTLV-III was identified, the WHO took its first serious step by establishing the Special Program on AIDS (SPA). Initially a small section of the organization's unit for infectious diseases, the SPA was soon made independent. In 1987, the WHO's World Health Assembly mandated the SPA to launch and supervise a "Global AIDS Strategy." In its statement, the Assembly commented boldly that the "assurance of global collaboration is of the highest priority, for AIDS cannot be stopped in any country until it is stopped in all countries" (WHO 1987, 5). The Assembly also granted the SPA the privilege of soliciting money directly from donors.[10]

As if to make up for his organization's delayed response, Mahler picked the very charismatic and impatient outsider, Jonathan Mann, to direct the new program. Mann had been working in what was then Zaire on the first research project to discover the presence of AIDS in Africa. At the WHO, Mann distanced himself immediately from what he called the "racist and speculative" debates about the alleged African origin of AIDS. Paradoxically, but in the way that would characterize his entire leadership, Mann accomplished this distance by throwing himself, and the WHO with him, into the middle of the fray. On the one hand, he defended Central and Eastern African countries by explicitly criticizing attempts to blame Africa for the disease and by shaming the wealthiest countries into giving relatively large amounts of money to the program. On the other hand, he put enormous pressure on the governments of Uganda, Kenya, and Tanzania especially to find out and report how many cases they had and to launch their own official AIDS-control programs. Meanwhile, Mann gathered medical and public health experts and gay, hemophiliac, and prostitute activists from all over the world to figure out what was and was not known about AIDS and how the WHO could help.

Mann wanted to create an essentially non-WHO-like program. He argued that to be effective, the SPA had to be centralized, top down, and vertical—that is, under his total and direct control and focused only on AIDS. Historically, the WHO had treated only smallpox[11] and, on occasion, malaria in this way. In general, the organization prided itself on the extent to which it devolved power to the regional offices and to which it championed broad-based, horizontally integrated "primary health care" and "wellness" approaches to health care development projects and policy (WHO 1978). According to Mann and Mahler, however, AIDS needed to be made visible to recalcitrant national governments. Visibility was produced by vertical and centralized programs in which scarce resources could be concentrated on the few risk groups responsible for spreading HIV first and most widely. As Manuel Carballo, the only one of Mann's close associates at the GPA still working at the WHO when I arrived in 1992, told me in an interview:

> When we set out the program, we felt that headquarters should assume a very important role; it should be the key driver, not only in developing the global but in actually working with countries. [It was necessary to take] conceptual, political, philosophical control —if you have one office, one philosophy is more easily propagated.[12]

In the name of global crisis, Mann not only bypassed the WHO's usual system of allocating funds to its various programs by soliciting money directly from donors, he also suspended the WHO's normal regionalized approach. In the case of Kenya and other African countries, this meant that the notoriously bureaucratic and slow-moving African Regional Office of the WHO headquartered in Brazzaville was left out of the financial and informational loop. Mann negotiated all policy and funding decisions directly with individual countries, first by visiting them and orchestrating the creation of national AIDS programs in each, and then by installing in them WHO representatives accountable only to Geneva.

While it had taken Mahler more than five years to respond at all seriously to AIDS, it took Mann less than three years to create a massive, highly visible, and by many accounts very successful campaign to stop it. In 1989, the "Special" Programme became the "Global" Programme on AIDS (GPA), a title that signified Mann's departure from the more indirect "internationalist" tradition of the WHO. The program saw its staff grow from three to more than 200 and its budget blossom from less than US$600,000 to $65.5 million (Mann, Tarantola, and Netter 1992,

520). The nongovernmental development organization Panos was one of a number of groups singing praises to Mann at the end of the decade:

> In just 18 months of unprecedented activity [between 1987 and 1989], Dr. Jonathan Mann, the programme's director, and his staff have firmly established WHO as the directing and co-ordinating agency of the global offensive against AIDS. Mann calls 1987, the year when the GPA was formally launched, "the year of global AIDS mobilization." At the centre of a whirlwind of country visits, consultations, meetings, briefings, conferences, speeches, interviews and articles, he and the programme staff have made an impact which is becoming evident in virtually every corner of the globe. (Panos 1989, 94)

There were things to be glad about. By 1988, overtly racist speculations about HIV's origin and about African sexual practices had largely stopped. We went from total uncertainty about where and how much the virus had spread to having relatively good estimates of how many people around the world were infected or at risk. Donor countries were cooperating with each other and coordinating their assistance to Africa. Many political leaders who had initially refused to admit that their people had anything to fear were finally making plans to control HIV within their borders.

Important dimensions of the crisis remained neglected, however. Despite his awareness of the plight of women in many poor countries and despite the presence in the WHO of female professionals urging the organization to deal more aggressively with women's health issues, Jonathan Mann did not seriously take up the "woman question" until the end of the first decade of the pandemic. Even then, the concern that gender inequality might put women at elevated risk was not at issue. Mann's GPA focused entirely on women as members of two categories of risk whose behaviors were considered to be important determinants of the spread of the epidemic: prostitutes and mothers.

Women as sex workers and women as mothers took center stage at the WHO in two conferences held in 1989: the Consultation on HIV Epidemiology and Prostitution held in Geneva in July and the International Conference on the Implications of AIDS for Mothers and Children in Paris that November. Beginning with these conferences, the problems of the spread of HIV by sex workers and mothers were defined internationally as two distinct and opposite poles of the transnational crisis.

Since the mid-1980s, prostitutes'-rights activists had been calling on Mann to respond to the growing tendency of governments, the media, and scientists to blame prostitutes for the heterosexual spread of HIV. Mann finally responded by convening a discussion among scientists, former prostitutes, current prostitutes, and prostitutes'-rights activists from all parts of the world. The meeting culminated in a statement that portrayed the spread of HIV via prostitution as a product of global political-economic inequality. Its chief point, and most radical departure from other UN statements on prostitution,[13] was that punitive laws against prostitution and discrimination against its practitioners at national and local levels were facilitating, if not entirely causing, the spread of HIV. The consensus statement published after the conference asserted:

> A major effect of legal and social restrictions on prostitution has been to generate low self-esteem among sex-workers and the belief that they cannot control their lives. Restrictive laws and adverse working conditions inhibit their ability to negotiate with clients and/or managers for adequate health care and safer sex practices. (WHO 1989, 3)

By contrast, the WHO's conference on The Implications of AIDS for Mothers and Children responded not to activists but to a new anxiety among demographers and international health experts. Perinatal HIV/AIDS was the latest and, it seemed, clearest proof that AIDS was a development crisis for Africa.[14] Infant HIV infection threatened the legitimacy and acceptance of the child-survival programs in which donor countries, particularly the United States, had heavily invested for decades.[15] The fear that mothers would soon learn that they might infect their babies by breastfeeding them and as a result undo years of struggle by experts to get women not to use baby formula was often expressed. There was fear that rumors that HIV had mutated from or, even worse, purposely been added to certain immunizations would undercut efforts to increase the numbers of pregnant women and children who received immunizations.

The document that came out of this meeting cast HIV infection in pregnant women as the result of the behaviors and attitudes of individual women, their communities, and their national governments. The document noted that because women's status often depends on their having children, women are likely to "resist" interventions to regulate their fertility. Meeting participants blamed "cultural attitudes and beliefs," "provider-client relationships," and "poverty and poor education" for women's low use of family planning (WHO 1990c, 3).

It is possible to see these two meetings and Mann's GPA as both progressive and regressive. They produced documents that challenged the narrow-mindedness of the medical community that had defined AIDS as a men's disease, denounced widespread and officially sanctioned discrimination against sex workers, and identified "women's empowerment" as an important tool in the struggle against HIV. It is also true, however, that Mann's approach to the problem of women and AIDS was premised on the old and too-familiar dichotomy between the whore as public—or, in this case, global—and the mother as domestic, in both senses of the word: national and private or family-related.

The existence of the binary opposition between mother and whore in international AIDS discourse has been noted by several feminist observers. Soon after these two meetings were over, Kathryn Carovano, a former staff member in the USAID's AIDS unit, wrote that by limiting discussions of women's position in the crisis to their purported relationship to one or the other of these dichotomous categories, international AIDS discourse misrepresents the realities of most women's lives (1991). She and others point out that many women face male demands for sex in exchange for material resources. Most of the same women are also likely to get pregnant and will be responsible for their children's health. Targeting some women as stigmatized, blameworthy prostitutes and others as honorable, victimized mothers ensures that AIDS education and interventions will not succeed.

Jonathan Mann's GPA laid over the whore-madonna duality an equally dichotomous distinction between the global and the national or domestic as arenas in which gender and sexual relations might be affected by AIDS-related policies. I have argued elsewhere (Booth 1999) that the drawing of this distinction in 1989 reflected a major tension in the GPA. On one side of this tension was Mann's own vision of a truly global program that had the power to define and enforce new (or perhaps highly reformed) social and political relations in the name of stopping AIDS—to create a sort of structural adjustment program for AIDS control paralleling the financial interventions of the International Monetary Fund. The consultation statement on prostitution was consistent with this global approach. It gave the WHO's support to a transnational movement of sex workers, called for the overhaul of national anti-prostitution laws, and confronted the hypocrisy of governments that depend for much-needed foreign exchange on the very sex workers they condemn.

The opposing view that the WHO ought to remain behind the scenes as a support and advisor to national governments was represented by many international health experts as well as by Hiroshi Nakajima, the man who in 1989 was poised to replace Halfdan Mahler as head of the WHO. These experts, some of whom participated in the Paris conference on HIV/AIDS in mothers and children and, subsequently, took over positions in the GPA after Mann resigned a year later, supported the more traditional "internationalist" approach of the pre-AIDS WHO. This ultimately triumphant strategy involves influencing national policy indirectly through "technical assistance" and expert advice. It appears to be benign, voluntary, and apolitical. It maintains that the nation-state, wherever located and however poor or rich, weak or strong, is the appropriate arbiter of what should be done to improve or protect its population's health.

As important as the WHO has been in shaping many African countries' responses to HIV/AIDS, the specific constructions of the AIDS crisis that emerged in Kenya and elsewhere are also affected by national political and economic factors. In March of 1992, I made a six-week preparatory trip to Nairobi. I was still trying to get permission from Kenya's National AIDS Control Programme (NACP) to do my research. On the suggestion of my Kenyan supervisor, I went to visit one of the important members of the National AIDS Committee, the government-appointed group in charge of defining and overseeing AIDS program activities in the country. When I told him that I was interested in studying the formation and effectiveness of Kenya's AIDS policies, he said, "What policies? Really, Kenya doesn't have any policy to speak of."[16] I was stunned, both about what he was saying and that he was saying it at all. I knew that the state's response to AIDS had so far been reactive, limited, and fairly quiet. It seemed to me, however, that the very existence of the NACP was evidence of policy. Even more shocking was that a member of the official AIDS policymaking body, apparently confidently and without embarrassment or fear of reprisal, admitted that the government had more or less done nothing about this by-now-enormous health crisis. I was also rather upset for myself; my research proposal depended on there being something policy-like to study. It did not seem that my chances of getting permission were very good. Two weeks later I left for Geneva, wondering if I would be able to return.

The words of this respected Kenyan scientist continued to trouble me long after I received permission to conduct my research. Could it be true that in the seven years since the first case of AIDS in Kenya was reported, President Moi, the ruling Kenya African National Union (KANU) party, the minister of health, or the parliament had issued no policy statement regarding AIDS or HIV? My working definition of "policy" was quite broad. I had used the term as what I hoped would be a palatable substitute for what I really meant but suspected would send up a red flag; that is politics, or the struggles, debates, tensions, and inequalities surrounding attempts to define and control heterosexual and perinatal transmission. I was not, therefore, confined to the study of official and public statements. Nevertheless, I did expect that there would be such things. So, of course, I started to look for them.

What I found, however, makes sense only in the context of the economic and political crises which were beginning to erupt when AIDS hit the headlines. With the end of the Cold War during the late 1980s, donors' willingness to continue financial support to indebted, economically stagnating, and newly strategically inconsequential African regimes had begun to wane. Donors justified such cuts in assistance by claiming that presidents such as Kenya's Moi were not "democratic" or "transparent," characteristics about which at least the United States had not been overly concerned before the fall of the Iron Curtain. Evidence that Kenya's ruling party was rather less than fully embracing and implementing the demands of the multiple structural adjustment programs imposed by the International Monetary Fund, moreover, was no longer officially ignored by the wealthy countries. The development rug was virtually overnight snatched from under Moi's feet just as AIDS was making its presence widely felt.

How did Kenya arrive at this set of economic, political, and health crises? When Kenya gained independence following more than a decade of violent struggle, its government "inherited institutions and conditions tending towards the intensification and perpetuation of existing economic inequalities, while at the same time [the] achievement of independence raised popular expectations for increased welfare" (Agonafer 1994, 108). Most former colonies faced a similar set of contradictory conditions. They also shared the problem of having been left economically underdeveloped in the wake of France and Britain's successful efforts to organize African economies to meet the needs of settlers in the colonies and of industrialists and middle-class consumers in the imperial center.

As former settler colonies, however, the "existing economic inequalities" in Kenya, Zambia (formerly Northern Rhodesia), and Zimbabwe (formerly Southern Rhodesia) were particularly great and especially difficult to eradicate. White settlers had taken or been given the most fertile land and created a large group of landless people. Kenya's response to this problem was to follow Britain's neoclassical economic plan based on private ownership of agricultural land, enormous wealth inequality, foreign direct investment, and an authoritarian state that put itself at the center of economic development.

For a while it looked like this strategy would work. Mulugeta Agonafer (1994) provides a good summary of Kenya's post-independence economic trends. He notes that Britain's continued support of Kenya through the 1960s and 1970s encouraged foreign investors to feel confident; Kenya became a favorite object of investors and donors during this period. The returns on this investment were considerable until the end of the 1970s. Export-oriented agriculture based mainly on the same large estates created by settlers and now run by the cronies of independent Kenya's first president, Jomo Kenyatta, was combined with urban-based import-substitution industrialization to achieve growth rates of nearly 6 percent for most of this period. This growth was very heavily dependent on foreign, mainly U.S. and British, investment; by 1972, foreigners owned 59 percent of the gross domestic product. The state itself owned or co-owned another 11 percent and provided 15 percent of formal-sector employment (Agonafer 1994, 118).

Not surprisingly, few foreigners were willing to criticize either the mounting corruption and autocracy of Kenyatta's regime or his lack of interest in redistributing the country's wealth. As Gîthînjî (2000) puts it, "stability" based heavily on the creation and maintenance of a militarized and repressive regime and on being a client of Britain and the United States in the fight against communism was the essential foundation for Kenya's economic growth. Even while they continued to repress local opposition with a heavy hand, Kenyatta and his successor Daniel arap Moi were praised by development experts because their regimes oversaw comparatively rapid improvements in literacy rates, life expectancy, child survival, and efforts to promote family planning.

Despite high rates of growth and favorable treatment by investors and donors, the Kenyan state was beset by problems common to many former British colonies. Because the British had trained very few Africans to run its bureaucracy, the state was left at independence with a cadre of young and inexperienced workers (Himbara 1994). By the end of the 1960s, Kenyatta was acknowledging that the economic and social infrastructures left behind by the British were in danger of collapsing as a result of a lack of skilled administrators (131).

The state responded to infrastructural problems with a two-pronged strategy. First, in order to attract members of Kenya's educated elite to the civil service, Kenyatta allowed public servants to own and benefit from unlimited amounts of property and to secure enormous profits from business (Himbara 1994, 122). Second, Kenyatta invited foreign experts to fill the gaps as consultants, advisors, and sometimes even permanent state employees.[17] The Canadian International Development Agency—many years later a key player in the planning and delivery of HIV/AIDS-related services through state-run clinics—sent a team to rebuild the ministry of finance in the 1970s and played a central role in designing the state's response to the oil crises of that decade

(148). This team was followed by a succession of advisors from the United Nations Development Programme (UNDP), the World Bank, and the USAID. These consultants supervised the state's less-than-enthusiastic attempts to implement its first structural adjustment program.

President Moi succeeded Kenyatta in 1978. Soon after, the so-called Kenya Miracle began to be exposed as a temporary trick. Within three years of taking office, Moi was facing severe economic problems. National and global economic downturns forced Moi to cut state expenditures. The cuts helped to spark a coup attempt in 1982 (Haugerud 1995). Because the air force officers leading the attempt very nearly succeeded and because their attempt was followed by increasing public dissent in Nairobi, Moi began working faster to concentrate power in his own hands (Grindle 1996, 67–68). By 1993, many top technocrats had left the civil service (124). This opened up even more space for foreign influence over policymaking. Despite this influence and growing pressures from the World Bank and the International Monetary Fund, Moi met inflation and declining economic growth with only half-hearted attempts to reduce public expenditures and rein in his efforts to fill his own coffers (72).[18]

By the end of the 1980s, political and economic problems had converged, catalyzed by a steep decline in coffee prices. Inflation and public dissent rose as economic growth slowed to zero and began to reverse. International agencies grew impatient with Moi's on again/off again response to structural adjustment (Grindle 1996, 73). Virtually overnight, the end of the Cold War rendered Kenya strategically irrelevant to the United States and Western Europe. The uncritical support that KANU had enjoyed from its foreign patrons for nearly thirty years ended simultaneously.

These conditions set the stage for increasing political dissent and repressive responses to it as well as the ever-louder silence about HIV that characterized the 1990s. Riots in Nairobi in 1990, led mainly by students and middle-class professionals, were aggressively put down; several dissenting church and government leaders were killed in mysterious accidents, and reports of severe human rights abuses leaked out of the country to international organizations. "By late 1992 and early 1993, Kenyans at all levels of society doubted the ability of the country to sustain its reputation for political stability and relatively effective management of political conflict" (Grindle 1996, 70). The collective decision of major donor countries to cut off US$350 million in aid to Kenya finally forced Moi to allow the formation of other political parties and to call for multiparty elections (Haugerud 1995).

Despite the best efforts of the American ambassador to support the

main opposition political party and despite unprecedented popular mobilization and public criticism of the regime, Moi won the 1992 elections. Both the foreign and the domestic bases of his support were much
weaker, however (Throup 1993). The early 1990s were characterized by
KANU's attempts to beef up what support Moi had left, encourage the
already-fragmented opposition to disintegrate further, and demonstrate
to the world that multipartyism in Kenya could lead only to chaos
(Haugerud 1995). The president forced many organizations of civil society, including Maendeleo ya Wanawake (MyWO), to become part of
the ruling party, effectively ending their nascent attempts to call for
reforms. Moi pursued a more deadly strategy when he encouraged members of his own ethnic group to foment a land war with mostly Kikuyu
farmers in the center of the country (Haugerud 1995, 38).

Not too surprising, given the state of its economic and political systems, Kenya's national campaign against AIDS got off to a rocky start.
Despite the fact that the first case of AIDS in a Kenyan who had not
traveled outside of Kenya had been diagnosed as early as 1984, there
was no official response until 1986. By this time, several U.S. and Canadian researchers were reporting that in Nairobi over 60 percent of
sex workers, nearly 15 percent of men diagnosed with STDs, and over
2 percent of pregnant women were HIV positive (Kreiss et al. 1986).

Much of the response that finally came took the form of righteous
nationalist denials and counteraccusations about AIDS as a disease of
Euro-American sexual perversion. Denial had its limits, however. When
newspapers reported that foreign tourists were canceling their plans to
visit Kenya because they were concerned about the safety of the country's blood supply, the understandably offended government quietly
called a meeting of senior health care officials and invited[19] the WHO's
Jonathan Mann to attend while it publicly continued to deny that there
was a problem.

Mann came to Nairobi armed with his standardized formula for a
national policy. Mann's plan was for all donors to contribute through
what the WHO called the National AIDS Programme (NAP) frame-
work and to be bound by the planning documents created collabora-
tively by the WHO and the individual country's NAP. The planning
documents would serve to demonstrate to donors that the WHO and the
government were committed to using their money for effective, scientifically informed control strategies. In order to ensure this, the GPA
established in each African national program a team of international
"experts," mostly epidemiologists and virtually all hailing from Europe or North America, to serve as "long-term advisers" to the nation-
als selected to run the NAP. The NAP was to be the site in which in-

ternational and national interests in AIDS were reconciled through a shared process of planning, financing, and applying technical knowledge (Mann, Tarantola, and Netter 1992).

What Kenya called its National AIDS Control Program (NACP) officially came into being on April 7, 1987. Following Mann's NAP model, it was to be an umbrella program incorporating all AIDS activities undertaken by the state, the private sector, nongovernmental organizations, and international donors and researchers (WHO 1988). It was to be supervised and coordinated by a committee whose members were to be Kenyan medical researchers appointed by the minister of health. Jonathan Mann and his chief of research, Manuel Carballo, represented the WHO in a meeting in Nairobi on February 24, 1987. At that time, Kenya's director of medical services signed a "Technical Services Agreement." This agreement committed the government to developing a program and committed the WHO to supplying "technical equipment and supplies for diagnostic centres" as well as funds for training health care personnel (Government of Kenya and WHO 1987, 2). This agreement set up the resource basis upon which the medium-term plan would be built. The medium-term plan served as both a contract between the state, the WHO, and donors and as policy which the staff of the NACP was supposed to implement.

Although most of Mann's staff had left the WHO by the time I arrived to do my fieldwork, Manuel Carballo, one of Mann's most important assistants, had stayed with the organization. I was able to talk to him about the creation of Kenya's NACP, in which he had played a key role. He described the process of getting the Kenyans to launch a program as not "too difficult." He explained to me that the relative ease resulted from two main preconditions: the existence of a well-trained group of medical researchers working in a state-subsidized research institute and the early research done on prostitutes by the Canadian and American microbiologists Frank Plummer and Joan Kreiss. "That initiative was very important in initiating the Kenyan AIDS program," Carballo insisted.[20]

Another GPA consultant who had been a part of the Kenya initiative had a somewhat different view of the start of the program. He was frustrated by the demands of Ministry of Health officials that the WHO deal first with the issue that most affected tourism: contaminated blood. He explained:

From the beginning [Ministry of Health people] were screaming only for blood [screening], while WHO's priority was prevention of sexual transmission. The tendency from the beginning was to develop sophisticated blood [screening]. If the sense of priorities was not developed, all available resources would go into sophisticated laboratories to screen screen screen and nothing else and then somebody would make a thesis on it and nobody would put money into information, education. Nobody [would] put money into condoms, and so on.[21]

I was unable to discover why the two WHO representatives had such different perceptions of the effort to get Kenya's NACP off the ground. I do know, however, that while Carballo had participated only in the initial meetings with state officials, the other consultant had been responsible for working out the NACP's first plan for AIDS control in subsequent meetings with lower-level Kenyan bureaucrats as well as with scientists and donor representatives. It is more than likely that, as usual, the devil lay in just such details.

In any case, the first medium-term plan for Kenya's AIDS-control program was completed just one month after Mann and Carballo's visit. I was told in Geneva and in Nairobi that the planning document and its successor were the closest things Kenya had to "AIDS policy." Its first paragraph, however, is more about Mann's main problem than about Kenya's actual HIV situation:

Kenya's cooperation with WHO and other donor institutions is based on the mutual recognition of the importance of positive cooperation aimed at overcoming the potential biases associated with this disease and the damaging steps and actions that these biases may cause that could rapidly undermine international confidence and cooperation. (Government of Kenya and WHO 1987, 2–3)

This paragraph names Mann's underlying motivation for establishing the NACP in Kenya and other African countries: the resolution of resolving "damaging" international conflicts through collaborative planning.

The document lays out what were then seen, at least by some, as the country's top priorities vis-à-vis controlling AIDS. According to the plan, the NACP's first concern was to ensure a safe blood supply. This focus was a response to attacks on Kenya's prestige in general and to questions about the safety of tourists and military personnel coming from the United States, Great Britain, and elsewhere in particular. The sexual transmission of HIV was of secondary importance. The plan's silence about sexual activity was nearly deafening. The government was apparently not ready to engage in a public discussion about sexuality or even to speculate about how many citizens had or would become infected.

Nevertheless, the planning document did suggest the need to educate the population about HIV and how it is and is not transmitted. A multilingual radio program to deliver information and education was proposed along with the creation of posters and pamphlets reminding citizens to "crush AIDS" (*kuvunja ukimwi*). Very little of the mass-education effort was devoted to explaining how Kenyans might protect themselves, however; there was no mention of condoms during the early years of AIDS control. The primary way in which the document confronted (hetero)sexual transmission was by briefly discussing the necessity of research on and interventions among two "risk groups": women prostitutes (sometimes confusingly referred to as "promiscuous" women) and male truckers who travel across national borders.

Funding the plan remained an issue. When the planning document had been written, sent back and forth between Geneva and Nairobi several times, and finally signed by both Mann and President Moi, donors pledged almost US$3.5 million to support the country's program through 1988.[22] This sum represented 92 percent of the total AIDS budget for the country. Although he was expected to contribute only US$300,000 (Government of Kenya and WHO 1987)—the remaining 8 percent—President Moi came up with nothing. It is not surprising that Kenyans came to see the NACP as an entirely foreign project. One GPA staff member made this clear when she reflected on the first few years of the program:

> [The donors] have done quite a lot. Even to formulate this first medium-term plan—it was sponsored by international organizations—through WHO. In one way or another, all the money that came to Kenya was channeled through WHO. International organizations or the international community has contributed a lot, especially in terms of financial assistance and sometimes in terms of expertise and in terms of exchange programs, seminars, conferences. Most of us have attended an international conference on AIDS at some time that was credited to one international organization or another; even those that are credited to WHO come from someone's pocket.[23]

Despite continuing pressure from GPA, that "someone" was never President Moi.

Officials in Geneva and Nairobi were divided in their views of the NACP's relative success and of the source of the various problems confronting it. The most positive assessment came from a Kenyan woman who had been an important staff member of the NACP since its inception. "The first two years here were exciting, challenging. In fact, all of the material you find here today was produced in 87–88. . . . At that time the donors were very generous; we had money and we mobilized a lot of people to do various things, produce materials for the general public."[24] Her account, although accurate, was probably also colored by a nostalgia born of the terrible decline in program funds and prestige she and the other NACP staff had been experiencing since 1990.

The contrast between her view and that of several observers both in Kenya and Geneva is startling. The program's critics focused on what they perceived to be either the ineptitude of the WHO's staff in the country or the corruption of the Kenyan bureaucrats running the NACP. Each NACP was supposed to have two staff members selected by Geneva to represent Mann locally. The "team leader" ran the program jointly with a national director, appointed by the minister of health. The "WHO administrator" was in charge of all monies and equipment that came to the national program from or via the GPA. Between 1988 and 1990, Kenya's NACP had three different team leaders and three different WHO administrators. In Geneva, one European WHO consultant who had worked in the WHO country office in Nairobi told me that the first WHO administrator alienated the Kenyan personnel. "He was behaving as a colonialist. He had a military background from the special forces in England, and he was acting as a captain."[25]

In Nairobi, a Kenyan social scientist who had consulted with the WHO agreed with this view and went on to complain about one of the team leaders. Because Denmark's contribution to the GPA's budget was earmarked to pay the salary of the team leader, Denmark selected that person. According to this consultant, the result was a disaster.

People were going wild. . . . We found that WHO's accountant [administrator] worked very closely with the [WHO] coordinator [team leader] and they were contracting without informing the [Kenyan] program manager. . . . How can you be a program manager and not know how much money you have? We say the program manager position has to be a very high one. WHO says it's a very junior doctor, so it has to be elevated. . . . The problem is administrative; who is to advise WHO? For heaven's sake, send us a qualified person. . . . If nobody from Denmark is qualified, we say "no." We were not amused. It is not the Africans who are squabbling; the lady is not qualified. It has to be someone with a wide experience—we can as well have ordinary Kenyans.[26]

Others at WHO headquarters aimed their criticisms at the state more generally, however. Several faulted the government for not creating a national budget specifically for AIDS. They and others also alluded frequently to state misuse of AIDS funds coming from outside the country. As one staff member diplomatically put it: "We have to send all the money for AIDS to the treasury and everybody knows it will be used for any other purposes. . . . AIDS officials won't control it. If the money is needed to pay teachers [it will go for that]. This is one of the obstacles mentioned in Kenya."[27] This problem, according to WHO consultants, continued to plague the organization's efforts to fight AIDS at least until 1995.

Nevertheless, some measures were taken. Jonathan Mann, with the help of a number of very committed Kenyans, transformed Kenya in the eyes of foreign donors. From a renegade, nationalist troublemaker where AIDS festered as a mysterious threat to white civilization, Kenya became a "needy" and relatively cooperative client of the GPA. In the form of the joint WHO-Kenyan NACP, Kenya could plan for, receive, and manage foreign resources. This, at least, was the image presented to the world. To some extent, the NACP was successful in getting a campaign started, despite official denials of the problem and refusals to discuss sexuality. But the NACP was beset by problems from the start. Like the population program and many other projects initiated by foreign concerns, AIDS control began and remained entirely dependent financially and scientifically on the WHO and foreign donors and researchers.

Because the WHO's AIDS program began to lose its vision and international support after 1990 and because donors started to withdraw their support from President Moi at about the same time, this dependence would put the prestige, and indeed the very survival, of the NACP in jeopardy. It would also, however, increase the authority and autonomy of foreign researchers as they began to design and implement their own HIV-control programs in Nairobi's public clinics.

In spite of his success, or perhaps because of it, Mann's attempt to use an *internationalist* ideology—the notion that the WHO can and should work through and "strengthen" the always-still-sovereign nation-state (Nicholas 1975)—to *globalize* policymaking—to create a single, standardized, worldwide movement under his own leadership—came to a crashing halt in 1990. In 1988, Halfdan Mahler died and Hiroshi Nakajima took over as the WHO's director-general. The leadership change, Nakajima's new "bureaucratic" style, and his lack of support from the United States and several other major donor countries hit Mann's GPA hard.[28] When, in the name of integrating AIDS programs (and hence the GPA) into the WHO's other programs, Nakajima blocked Mann from receiving more than $100 million that donors had committed to AIDS control, Mann and most of his staff resigned.

Jonathan Mann made his criticisms of the new regime both clear and public. In his resignation speech, he said that it had become "crystal clear to me that to remain in the program would be to preside over the dismantling of the most important elements of the program, both from a programmatic aspect and from a philosophic aspect" (quoted in Mann and Kay 1991, S225). Suiting his actions to Mann's words, Nakajima's new director of the GPA quickly reduced the scope of its work, created a more traditional hierarchy, and devolved much greater power (and financial responsibility) back to the regional offices from which Mann had taken it. The GPA's largest donors responded by cutting their contributions to the program and giving more of their HIV/AIDS-control dollars to other agencies.[29]

The new head of the GPA, Michael Merson, expanded the managerial dimension of technical assistance. Unlike Mann, he focused on strategies that at least appeared to have the potential for making national programs more cost effective and less dependent on the WHO and donors. He regionalized the AIDS programs, putting them in line with the WHO's other activities; this move decreased the authority, autonomy, and, probably, effectiveness of both headquarters and national programs but silenced the complaints of the heretofore-ignored staff at the WHO's Regional Office for Africa.

Merson's uncharismatic and international-politics-as-usual style gave a push to a trend that had already begun in the late 1980s. Rich countries' donor agencies, new and old international nongovernmental organizations, universities, and multinational pharmaceutical companies were beginning to bypass the WHO and intervene directly in HIV/AIDS projects in Africa and elsewhere. Officially, the GPA described such changes as inevitable and even positive (WHO 1990d). The world, Merson argued, had realized that fighting AIDS required interventions in more than just health care; it was just as much, if not more, an economic problem as it was a medical crisis (WHO 1992a). In countries such as Kenya, the GPA now asserted, the "vertical" approach to AIDS (one that focused on a single disease) and hence the single-organization strategy that Mann had designed was too expensive and inefficient.

According to Merson, AIDS was no longer (if it ever was) a global disease; it was now a disease of "developing" countries. Merson estimated, correctly as it has tragically turned out, that these countries would account for 90 percent of all HIV infections in 2000. At a 1991 conference in Senegal, Merson explained why:

Why is Africa so hard hit by the pandemic? One reason is poverty. I submit that poverty has made this continent vulnerable to infection, by fostering political instability and conflict that drives people from their homes, by forcing men to leave their families in search of work, by making prostitution a survival strategy for women and children. And, tragically, having grown out of this poverty, AIDS completes the vicious circle by worsening it in turn. Poverty breeds AIDS breeds poverty. (Merson 1991, 4)

In a subsequent press release, Merson substituted the term "development" for poverty: "*The* obstacle to controlling AIDS is heterosexual transmission and therefore heterosexual risk behaviors; because most of these people are or will live in poor countries, the economics of the epidemic have to be addressed now. AIDS is fundamentally a *development* crisis" (WHO 1992a). According to Merson, "African AIDS" is not about global inequalities as it was, partly at least, for Mann. "These people," heterosexual Africans, live in poor places. Thus, Merson concludes, AIDS in Africa is about poverty and (a lack of) development at the national level. Development is about national economics. Thus, in Africa (and, apparently, nowhere else) AIDS is about domestic economics; AIDS is just one more local development problem.

Another change from Mann's more global orientation was a bit more surprising. Merson's global AIDS strategy paid considerable attention to women qua women. In 1990, he issued several press releases in honor of World AIDS Day, the focus of which Mann had already decided would be women and AIDS. The press releases asserted that to stop AIDS it was essential to "empower" women politically, economically, and culturally, since "women are especially vulnerable to HIV infection because of their generally subordinate role in family and society . . . [which] has the effect of restricting women's ability to protect themselves from sexual transmission of HIV because they often have little autonomy and little say about sexual matters" (WHO 1990a, 2). One of the six major goals of the new strategy Merson submitted to the World Health Assembly in 1992 was to reduce women's vulnerability to HIV infection "through an improvement of women's health, education, legal status, and economic prospects" (WHO 1992a, 1). It seemed that the WHO was finally defining women's health as an issue in its own right. Radical for the typically conservative WHO, and especially for Merson, the statement seemed to give hope to those feminists who had started to pay attention to the epidemic.

As I later learned from my interviews with the GPA staff who were in various ways dealing with women's issues, these statements were the result of a great deal of prodding from feminists working in Scandinavian donor agencies and in the GPA itself. Denmark in particular had remained supportive of the GPA but was applying a lot of pressure on Merson to stay on the cutting edge of AIDS politics. Because of this pressure, Merson launched an effort to design what he called a plan of action and what the mostly women staff members at the GPA called a strategy. A group of about ten GPA staff members along with an expert from the maternal and child health and the reproductive health units started meeting together to design this strategy.

Over time, it became clear to me and to at least some of the participants that there was no consensus on just what the WHO should or could do about gender and sexual inequalities around the world. According to Kathleen Cravero, the head of the group responsible for developing the strategy, the effort to create a document listing what the WHO should do to deal with the problems faced by women "is a chance to make [HIV/AIDS] more relevant to women for the reasons that the ministries of health—many—are controlled by doctors, many of whom are men. We are looking at the specific problems of women and AIDS."[30] She was, however, only moderately optimistic about the effect such a strategy would have on the WHO's work.

> We haven't asked [GPA staff] to do anything yet. If you ask, "Do you support an integrating strategy for women?," 99.9 percent will say, "Yes." Oh, occasionally someone will say it's divisive; we shouldn't separate women. But I am not impressed with general support. I'll be impressed when documents are looked over to see how sensitive [they are to women's issues]; then I'll be impressed.[31]

At the time we met, she believed that her group's efforts to get the project going had so far had little impact.

When the "women's internal working group" met in December 1992 to discuss the strategy document, disagreements between members over just what the WHO should do and how became clear. Some participants argued that the strategy should identify individual behaviors to be changed and suggest related reforms to national health programs. They argued that improving women's access to sexually transmitted disease treatment, offering better contraceptives, reducing the stigmatization of condoms, and making guidelines to help counselors cope with a woman's "horror of infecting her baby," as one participant put it, would help women deal with HIV/AIDS.[32] They did not think that the

WHO could or should explicitly address, let alone change, macrolevel problems of inequality embedded in laws, labor relations, family structures, and, more generally, ideologies (Booth 1999).

Others involved in developing the women-and-AIDS strategy wanted to try a different approach. They argued that the GPA's mission to promote empowerment required it to intervene actively and decisively in social and political relations. They urged the group to demand, for example, that states decriminalize prostitution and allow sex workers to form labor unions. They also suggested that the GPA go over the laws on rape and domestic violence in each nation receiving WHO support. If a country did not have adequate protections, it was proposed, the WHO should pressure the government directly and even consider withholding funds (Booth 1999). In order to put such pressure on governments, however, the GPA would have had to continue growing and functioning the way that Jonathan Mann had envisioned: as a top-down, highly visible, and financially centralized global force.

It is not surprising that in the end the less radical strategy of maintaining the WHO's apparently apolitical "advisory" role won out at the GPA. The organization's leadership had already rejected Jonathan Mann's vision, which meshed more with the macrolevel, top down, and explicitly political (if not the explicitly feminist) strategy suggestions. Most of the women's internal working group's members were aware that neither Merson nor Nakajima would support a strategy that demanded major social transformations. Ultimately the strategy document took the form of a list of suggested strategies from among which national programs might (or might not) choose when planning their own campaigns. For example, one of the staff people at GPA headquarters said that it was important that African countries recognize that women are often put at risk by their male partners' decisions to have multiple sexual partners rather than by the women's own sexual behavior. The inclusion of such a recognition was listed as a possible way to "implement" the women-and-AIDS strategy at the national level. The guidelines do not demand national adherence nor do they reference any global standards for women's rights or recognize the importance of women's social movements (WHO 1993b).

Several of the women's internal working group's participants calling for a more interventionist and directive policy soon resigned or were fired from the GPA. When I was in Geneva, many of those who had come to work at the GPA because they admired Jonathan Mann's approach were deeply disillusioned and frustrated at what they saw as the "red tape" and conservative bureaucratic style of Merson. For some of them, the outcome of the women-and-AIDS strategy conflict was simply the last straw.

By the end of 1992, discussions were under way at the United Nations about whether the WHO should remain the lead agency in the fight against AIDS or if the UNDP should take over. The UNDP is directly under the control of the UN secretary-general. It has a much broader and more flexible mandate than the GPA. It is also obviously much more oriented toward "development," which was the rubric under which Nakajima and Merson wanted to fit AIDS. The future of the GPA was clearly in jeopardy. Merson apparently did not perceive this to be a bad thing, however. It seemed, in short, that Merson intentionally presided over his own agency's demise.

Meanwhile, back in Kenya, AIDS politics were continuing to provoke local and international debates. As rates of HIV infection in the so-called general population rose to between 13 and 20 percent, the Kenyan government announced that it had discovered Kemron, a "cure" for HIV/AIDS. European and American scientists' dismissal of both the drug's efficacy and Kenya's claims to have discovered it were quickly taken up by African Americans and Africans as proof that non-Africans did not care if Africans died. The dismissals also made it clear to many African Americans and Africans that white folks believed Africans were too stupid to develop a cure by themselves. Some HIV-infected African Americans called Kemron the Afrocentric drug and flew to Nairobi to pay exorbitant prices for it. The WHO quickly issued a press release stating that Kemron was really a low-dose antiretroviral drug invented by a Japanese and American research team. Apparently the team had sent the drug to Kenyan laboratories only for final testing. The drug, the WHO claimed, had already been found to be ineffective (WHO 1993a).

In the background, Kenya's NACP struggled more quietly to do something about the crisis. Its staff was plagued by structural, personal, and financial problems, however. Mann's effort to create a program that would be accountable to the WHO and through it to donors produced a dual institutional structure in Kenya and in other African countries. On the one hand, the program was a part of the national health bureaucracy. It brought under government control desperately needed resources for laboratory development, drug purchasing, and personnel training. Foreign donors, represented by the WHO's staff in Kenya, were nervous about whether the government was capable of using these resources in what the WHO deemed appropriate ways. On the other hand, the program was part of the GPA and had been directly associated with Jonathan Mann and his assistants. The state employees were at best ambivalent about and often hostile to the foreign staff who were supposed to "guide" and "strengthen" them. These relationships gave shape to the local relations in which Nairobi's nurses found themselves at the time of my fieldwork in the clinics.

The second medium-term plan, which was drafted in 1992, represented a collaborative attempt to address these conflicts.

> As many as 300,000 new adult and 115,000 new paediatric AIDS cases may develop during the next five years. This will have major effects not only on the individuals, their families and health system, but also on the communities and the society as a whole. The major impacts expected include: [an] overburdened health system which will overstretch the health budget; drainage of community resources; disintegration of family structures; an increasing number of orphans and abandoned children; worsened status of women; decline in economic growth and its implications for national security. (Government of Kenya and WHO 1992, 12)

Based on this assertion, the second medium-term plan called for an institutional restructuring. The NACP was to be reorganized in such a way that all government ministries were involved in planning and implementing control efforts. According to the plan, HIV/AIDS is, or should be, a matter of relevance and concern to all sectors of government. The plan called for the creation of an "intersectoral board" that would oversee the AIDS program and expected that representatives from all government ministries would participate in the workshops where the plan would be made operational (iii).

The document also listed new goals for HIV/AIDS control. The planners gave much more attention to women and babies than in the first medium-term plan, although they did not actually call for government intervention in gender inequality. A major goal of the second plan was to reduce the transmission of HIV to infants (11). The plan stated that reducing perinatal transmission would require lowering HIV prevalence among pregnant women from 10 percent (which was already an undercount) to 7.5 percent in five years (23). The program was to accomplish this by targeting women 15 to 24 years old who come to public clinics for prenatal care and giving them STD treatment and HIV counseling. By emphasizing the reduction of perinatal transmission, the second medium-term plan addressed a growing concern among women worldwide; that is, that their risk of getting HIV creates for them a distinct and serious biological and social problem, the possibility of being unable to bear healthy children. Because low-income women's status and social security depend on their ability to bear children and to see them become adults, the problem of mother-to-child HIV transmission has to be understood not only as a disaster for infant mortality rates but also as a gendered economic, social, political, and cultural crisis of enormous significance.

It is rather surprising that the plan also referred explicitly, albeit vaguely, to the problem of a "worsened status of women" (12). The inclusion of this apparent problem in the list of expected "main effects of the HIV/AIDS problem" about which nothing can be done is less surprising. To have instead identified "women's status" (or, of course, more radically, gender inequality) as a cause of the epidemic would have required the planners to include improving women's status in the list of policy interventions.

Finally, the document called for the dual recognition that "by far the commonest mode of transmission in Kenya is sexual transmission" (10). This statement might seem so obvious as to be unnecessary. But neither the first planning document nor any official government statements about HIV/AIDS prior to this had acknowledged that HIV is primarily sexually transmitted. According to the GPA consultant who led the meetings in which this document was produced, the willingness of the participants to state this and their insistence that it be included in the document represented something of a sea change in official attitudes.

The plan also asserted that the risk of infection incurred by an individual whose "partner [is] having multiple sexual partners" is one of the most important "elements . . . identified to play a role in sexual transmission" (10). According to the WHO consultant who worked on this in Nairobi during the planning stage, this statement was a radical departure for the Kenyan team. Although the document did not specify which individuals were most likely to be put at risk in this way, the consultant explained to me that the reference to having a partner who has multiple partners "clearly" spoke to Kenyan women's distinct vulnerability to HIV. "Most" Kenyan women, he asserted, were put at risk of infection not by their own sexual behaviors but by those of their husbands or male partners. This consultant and, apparently, the other participants involved in the planning process, believed that Kenyan women were both consistently monogamous and sexually powerless. In their view, policies on the treatment and counseling of women had to be redesigned to address (if not redress) this powerlessness.[33]

Radical or not, the second medium-term plan was not endorsed by the government. The minister of health's inaction gave donors an official reason for refusing to hold a "donor mobilization" meeting, the calling of which requires the mutual understanding that an endorsed plan is equivalent to policy. The result of this and of the fact that the state had still not created a separate budget line for AIDS was that the NACP was broke and unable to respond to requests for support and assistance. Both the prestige and the capacity of the program declined. One Kenyan staff member gave me an example: "We were completely out of test kits [for blood screening]. The newspapers put blame on the government for being unable to supply test kits. You feel it all the time. The district and mission hospitals blame the program all the time if there are no test kits."[34]

Another longtime member of the Kenyan staff complained that she was unable to start anything new. "A major difficulty is that we can't plan on a continuous basis when we don't know where the resources are coming from. If we could, we could plan—what have we done and not done . . . even one-quarter of the activities . . . [but] the money is not available."[35] I was asked by a number of Kenyans who knew that I was studying the AIDS program whether the program was "doing anything." The view that the NACP had become irrelevant seemed widespread among Kenyans.

Officials at the WHO in Geneva essentially agreed with this view. Several commented that they were just waiting for the government to endorse the plan so that they could hold a meeting with the donors and get some money committed to the NACP. From their perspective, the problem lay in state corruption or, as one official put it more diplomatically, the lack of a "sound mechanism to channel external funds."[36]

The WHO team leader in Nairobi believed that the problem was linked to the broader tensions between donors and Moi that had been in the making for some time. The donors, she said, "really want a new political situation. They are not satisfied with how much the MOH [Ministry of Health] is working, and that really affects most of what we do." She went on: "The government has a special relationship to donors now. Some of them, led mainly by the U.S., are trying to push for change in the political system and that's not nice for the government to involve those people [i.e., the government does not want to have those people participate in policymaking]. They see AIDS as a sensitive issue relating to their economy, to the image of the country."[37]

Kenyans in the national program blamed the WHO, and specifically the changes that Merson had ushered in, for the loss of donor support. As one staff member put it:

In early 1989 it was changing. [People at the WHO] were thinking they wanted the program to run the way the Ministry of Health is run. But that's why we established this program, to minimize the red tape of the government. Because of the change [in administration], the money the donor community gave us to give out to people who were potential implementers went down. We did a bit of work, but it went down down down.[38]

In January 1993, the National AIDS Program was still a visible institution, housed in a bright yellow house with a fence, a guard, and a few white Land Rovers with the WHO seal on the side. It had, however, virtually ceased to function as a policymaking entity. A number of "needs assessment" reports lay on tables collecting dust. The new consultant on orphans waited, and waited, for her first assignment. The WHO team leader kept busy collecting HIV seroprevalence data from clinics around the country and fixing the often broken computers that were supposed to analyze the data. No one seemed to know to what use this information would be put. There was, quite simply, no money. With the money had gone the staff's morale. There was an air of expectancy, of hope that the minister of health would sign the second medium-term plan and that donors would begin to fund their work again. But optimism on that score was not high.

This state of things seemed to me to reflect quite well the more general political climate in Nairobi at the time. In December of 1992, President Moi won the country's first multiparty elections since 1964. Many Kenyans who had hoped that these elections would usher in a truly new kind of government were deeply disappointed and alienated. The opposition, which was now at least recognized, had nonetheless largely lost its critical edge; many opposition politicians had become engaged in the same old game of ethnic politics and vote-buying. A civil war escalated in the central part of the country, the region many of Nairobi's middle-class citizens call home. Kenyans were anything but hopeless; as always, grassroots organizations were active on many fronts. But energy had waned. And there was no end in sight to the country's worst-ever economic crisis. In this context, the work of the foreign researchers who are the subject of the next chapter and of the nurses working for them whom we visit in chapter 5 took on greater significance. For the foreseeable future, the AIDS crisis was theirs to define.

Four

"High-Frequency Transmitters" and Invisible Men

In 1989, I began contacting people in Nairobi and Geneva to ask whether my plan to study "AIDS policy" and urban women was likely to be acceptable to the government. I knew that to study national policy I would have to get permission from the Office of the President in Nairobi. I also knew that in Kenya at that time a study of AIDS as a social and political issue (rather than as a strictly medical one) was not likely to be among that office's most appealing research projects. My dissertation advisor suggested that I write to Dr. Elizabeth Ngugi at the University of Nairobi and ask for advice about how to negotiate the clearance process. He had just met Dr. Ngugi in Geneva at a WHO workshop on HIV/AIDS in Mothers and Children. I wrote to her and received a very welcoming letter inviting me to join the Department of Community Health at the University of Nairobi as her student. She generously offered to help me gain research clearance for the project.

This letter began what became for me both a productive and problematic relationship. Through Dr. Ngugi's interest in my project and her willingness to assist me, I was linked and tacitly beholden to the Canadian-led multinational team of medical researchers who had hired Dr. Ngugi to help them establish what was eventually referred to as the "Nairobi cohort" of sex workers. Because Dr. Ngugi had become an indispensable part, indeed a leader, of the research team, all of the foreign and Kenyan students associated with her, including myself,[1] were in some way connected to the team. I made good friends among the students and staff of the research project. I enjoyed a free dinner at a fancy Nairobi restaurant and more than one party with them. I got to ride in their Land Rover. Through Dr. Ngugi I eventually received research clearance for my project. I was also given letters of introduction and access to clinics by virtue of my (never fully defined) association with the project. All of this was, of course, wonderful. Without this help, my project would not have been possible.

As I worked in the clinics, interviewed national and international bureaucrats, and read the medical literature on AIDS in Africa, however, I became aware of what the authority of this group to which I had attached myself meant for policy constructions of Kenyan women and for the local practices based on those constructions. This project trained the nurses I interviewed; created and put into effect the diagnostic, treatment, and prevention regimens those nurses were trying to implement; and bought the drugs and blood-testing equipment the nurses were using. It was this project that positioned nurses simultaneously as data collectors and policy innovators, as agents of multinational science and as agents of the state. I decided that in order to understand how, why, and with what implications Kenya had made urban working-class women's sexuality the central problematic of the AIDS crisis, I had to dissect—very critically, as it has turned out—the work of the very people who had made my research possible in the first place. It is therefore with both ambivalence and trepidation that I undertake in this chapter what literary scholars refer to as a close, critical reading of the most important texts this research project produced from 1980 up through the time my fieldwork ended in 1994.

The Nairobi STD/AIDS research group, as it came to be called, has been both prolific and influential. They are responsible for nearly 40 percent of all English-language articles on HIV in Kenya and over two-thirds of all articles published on HIV or STDs in Kenyan women since the HIV epidemic began. More important, theirs is the only research on HIV in Kenya that has been published in two of the most important and influential English-language biomedical journals, the *New England Journal of Medicine* and the *Journal of the American Medical Association*. Half of the articles on AIDS in Kenya published during the first decade of the crisis by *The Lancet*, Britain's most important medical journal, were written by this team as well. Frank Plummer, who has directed the program since 1981, also co-authored one of the most influential early articles on the international epidemiology of HIV (Piot et al. 1988). This article was published in the American journal *Science*, which is read widely among both scientists and the lay public. Various members of the team have written chapters in the recent edition of the book generally considered to be the definitive English-language source of information about sexually transmitted diseases (Holmes, Sparling, and Wasserheit 1998).[2] According to WHO officials, the research group played a central role in the negotiations between the WHO and the Kenyan government over the creation of a National AIDS Program, which was used as a model for designing other such programs elsewhere. Recently, the group initiated one of the world's most important investigations into the possibility of an HIV vaccine. A U.S. company has even produced a documentary about the group's work among Nairobi's prostitutes (Krotz 1999).

The story of the Nairobi project begins in the late 1970s with two outbreaks of a sexually transmitted disease (STD) in Manitoba, Canada. The disease, known as chancroid, is rare in North America. As a result, very little was known about chancroid's microbiological causes or symptoms at the time these outbreaks occurred. Alan Ronald of the University of Manitoba wanted to learn more (Ronald et al. 1991). To do so, however, required finding a place with a larger population of people with the disease. It is not clear to me precisely why Ronald chose Nairobi to do further research on chancroid. In a history of the project up through the 1980s, Ronald and others who later joined the team indicate that the existence of Casino, the long-lived STD clinic in downtown Nairobi, was part of Nairobi's appeal (Ronald et al. 1991). The group's first publication claimed that over a three-year period in the 1970s, Casino saw more than 20,000 patients with genital ulcers (Nsanze et al. 1981, 378).

The project had both a medical research and a health care development mandate from the start. When the man whose name would soon be inseparable from the project took it over from Ronald in 1981, he did so with funds from the science and international development arms of the Canadian state. Frank Plummer got grants from the Medical Research Council of Canada, the Canadian International Development Research Centre and, eventually, the Canadian International Development Agency (CIDA). The two arms of medical research and health development became further entwined as the project became more international. In 1983, the WHO made the Nairobi offices of the project a "collaborating center" for STD research. This move gave the project international status, access to people and resources at the WHO, and a certain level of responsibility for training local scientists and improving the research infrastructure in Kenya. The team was joined by several researchers from the University of Antwerp in Belgium and from the University of Washington in Seattle.

Ronald and Plummer also recruited several Kenyan researchers, including Dr. Elizabeth Ngugi and several experts based at the Kenyan Medical Research Institute (KEMRI). Many of the Kenyan researchers have been first or second authors on papers published by the team in major U.S. and British journals. The Canadians also made it possible for a number of Kenyan scientists to present research at international STD and AIDS conferences. KEMRI's support doubtlessly lent the program some degree of national legitimacy and state tolerance; the institute enjoyed President Moi's favor.

Although Alan Ronald arrived in Nairobi in the 1970s, it was not until 1986 that this group caught the attention of the medical world beyond Nairobi and the WHO's STD unit. Tragic as the epidemic has been for all people, biomedicine's discovery of AIDS and of how it spreads has given this project (and many other heretofore low-status STD projects) an enormous boost, propelling its directors and its data onto the pages of the world's most prestigious medical journals and even, occasionally, of several major U.S. and Western European newspapers. The University of Washington team, including internationally recognized STD expert King Holmes, "identified the spread of HIV among the prostitute cohort" that Plummer and Ngugi had been following for more than two years (Ronald et al. 1991, 339). Together the Seattle and Manitoba groups published the *New England Journal of Medicine* article that announced the arrival in East Africa of the virus then called HTLV-III. This article put Nairobi and this research team on the AIDS research map. A subsequent article in the very prestigious journal *Science* built heavily on this early research and has had a lasting impact on AIDS research around the world. The multinational team served, moreover, as the key liaison and support for the efforts of the WHO's Global Programme on AIDS to launch an AIDS-control program in Kenya.

Money followed the researchers' discovery of AIDS. The project's original funding agencies were joined by the European Economic Community (EEC), the U.S. National Institutes of Health, and the American Foundation for AIDS Research, as well as CIDA and several private foundations and pharmaceutical companies (Ronald et al. 1991, 339). The researchers had their own building erected within the University of Nairobi's medical school. Soon, more Canadian, American, European, and Kenyan students signed up to work on the project.

The team has made several important contributions to our understanding of both HIV transmission and the improvement of health care services, particularly for women in Nairobi. Most significant, they have made us aware of the importance that treating conventional (but often-ignored) STDs plays in preventing and controlling HIV. By the end of the 1980s, they had provided important evidence supporting an STD "co-factor" theory to explain why HIV was spreading so fast among African heterosexuals. The researchers improved, indeed often started, STD treatment and counseling services in many of Nairobi's clinics.

They have worked hard to convince the government of the importance of STD treatment.[3] Their efforts have benefited many women who might well have suffered serious long-term consequences from untreated syphilis, gonorrhea, chancroid, or other diseases. The researchers have expanded the local awareness of STDs in Kenya and probably given many women and men reason to attend to their sexual health.

Unlike many other foreign researchers, Plummer and his group have not done "safari research," that is, research to make a quick discovery followed by a total exit. They have stayed, trained many Kenyans, built or renovated several clinics and laboratories, developed some interesting peer-education counseling projects (Ngugi et al. 1996), and secured funding for a deeply troubled and resource-poor health care system. The Belgian scientists on the team have also added a great deal to our still-limited understanding of how HIV affects pregnant women and newborns. It is difficult to overestimate the importance of these contributions to the health of a country facing severe economic as well as epidemiological crises.

Nevertheless, guiding this research and the policies and interventions based on it is a scientifically and sociopolitically problematic model of heterosexuality in Kenya. Because it has been so central not only to the projects that I studied in Nairobi's clinics but also to the development of medical and policy discourse on HIV/AIDS in Africa more broadly, it is crucial to understand how the model is described, what the data is to support it, and, perhaps most critical, what social and biological dimensions of HIV transmission it leaves out.

My analysis here is influenced by feminist and anti-imperialist critiques of the system and language of the science that gained ascendancy in Western Europe and its white majority colonies during the sixteenth century and is now hegemonic worldwide.[4] This particular mode of thinking about, seeing, and explaining the world is based on the now very widely accepted premise that the knowledge (what we usually call facts) produced according to its rules, within its institutions, and by the people who are trained to do it is objectively true. In other words, when produced correctly within this system, scientific facts are true for all people, at all times, and under any social, political, or economic conditions. By its own definition, scientific thought—unlike every other form of thought—is unaffected by its producers' race, class, gender, sexuality, or relationship to the project of colonization; it is, in short, mere coincidence, albeit a happy one for colonizers and scientists, that this system emerged at the same moment, among the same people, and in the same place that the project of exploring, conquering, and dividing up the world beyond Europe was formed.

Radical scholars (including some scientists) have repeatedly demonstrated that this central assumption is fundamentally flawed. Science's critics argue that just like every other mode of thought, modern scientific thought at a minimum reflects and at the extreme produces and entrenches the social conditions and relationships in which it was born and which became the supreme system of knowledge production. Feminist critiques of science have focused on showing us how what counts as objective scientific knowledge, including biomedical knowledge, reproduces gender inequality; that is, men's privilege and the oppression of women and transgendered people. Feminists have also argued that science perpetuates heterosexuals' privilege and the oppression of all other forms of sexual expression. Anti-imperialist scholars have demonstrated that the simultaneous emergence of modern science and modern imperialism was not coincidental; science has been a crucial tool for making the European conquest of Africa, Latin America, and Asia both possible and apparently legitimate. Likewise, conquest provided scientists with the raw materials they needed to make modern science the most expansive system of thought, apparently able to classify and explain everything on the planet. When combined, the work of these critics reveals that what we often accept as scientifically and therefore objectively true is instead a historically and geographically particular story told from the point of view of the relatively small group of people who have the most political, economic, and intellectual power and of the much larger group who have been trained by them.

Anti-imperialist and feminist critics of modern science go farther than simply showing that scientific knowledge is no more (or less) objective or free from the effects of history and social relations than other modes of thought, however. They argue that the false claim that scientific knowledge is objective has legitimized its domination over and suppression of other systems of thought or worldviews by successfully masking its partiality (and the partiality of its producers). Modern science's triumph lies in its ability to wield the magic wand of objectivity and make what are actually changeable relations of inequality—between women and men, heterosexual and homosexual, rich and poor, colonized and colonizer, researcher and researched, doctor and patient—appear to be fixed, natural, inevitable, universal, and eternal truths.

My aim in this chapter is to use the published articles that came out of the Nairobi HIV/STD Project in the 1980s and early 1990s as an important example of how a particular view of Africa, African women, and African sexuality is embedded in and naturalized by apparently objective scientific research on an extremely serious health crisis. I am not suggesting that the individual scientists involved in this project or the

Kenyans they trained to help them are intentionally producing racist and sexist accounts of AIDS in Africa. On the contrary, I argue that the doubtlessly good intentions of most of the project staff and of the majority of AIDS researchers working in sub-Saharan Africa are foiled by a scientific language that is designed to hide and thereby reinforce both its own particularity and the unnatural, noninevitable, and political character of the conditions it is studying.

I am not arguing that the scientists on the Nairobi team are unusual or deviant. Their research is not only consistent with accepted normal science, it is also probably some of the best and most immediately useful of the vast amounts of biomedical knowledge about HIV being produced in Africa and elsewhere. The literature that has come out of this project is important precisely because it is typical as well as abundant and influential. It is also important, and important to understand, because it puts into the controlled, rule-bound, and globalizing language of what is widely referred to as "normal" science the complex, messy, and contradictory relations of everyday life in the clinics where I was able to work.

The Model

The first, and arguably still the most influential, article on AIDS that the multinational research group published provides some of the broad outlines of this model. The article appeared in the widely read and respected *New England Journal of Medicine* in 1986 and has been cited nearly 400 times since. It begins by reasserting one of the central premises of the "African paradigm": the presumption that African AIDS is a wholly different phenomenon from the epidemic that had by then taken shape in the United States:

> The acquired immunodeficiency syndrome (AIDS) has been occurring in epidemic form in Central Africa since the late 1970s. The epidemiology of AIDS in Africa differs from that of AIDS in the United States. Whereas homosexual activity and parenteral transmission account for the majority of cases in the United States, transmission through heterosexual activity appears to predominate in Africa. (Kreiss et al. 1986, 414)

It continues by increasing the distance between the two epidemics. The article's most important conclusion is that neither North Americans nor Europeans were responsible for bringing the virus to Kenya:

The source of the AIDS virus epidemic in Nairobi must remain speculative, but our data support the hypothesis of transcontinental spread from Central Africa rather than introduction of the virus by visitors from Europe or North America. None of the prostitutes in the low socioeconomic class had had sexual contact with a non-African. (417)

This introduction to the researchers' findings that over 60 percent of Nairobi's prostitutes were infected with HIV must be interpreted in light of the international debates and the climate of hostility, blame, and denial surrounding AIDS in the mid-1980s. The article does not explicitly reference the political debates over whether AIDS originated in Africa, whether tourists should cancel their safaris, whether Kenyan students abroad should be sent home to protect a nation from AIDS, or whether "perverted" Euro-Americans or "promiscuous Africans" were the more culpable. Nevertheless, it does speak to the issues with which the WHO's Jonathan Mann was struggling at the very same time the data for the 1986 article was being analyzed. The discovery of HIV antibodies in Kenyan women, of course, directly challenged Kenyan president Daniel arap Moi's denials that AIDS could be found in Kenya. The comment and the data the researchers provide to support it also dismiss Moi's claims that the virus must have originated outside of Africa. Moreover, the article predicts that HIV will continue to spread not only in Kenya but to other African countries as well.

Of longer-term significance for the politics and policies of AIDS, however, is the way that the authors present the epidemiological scenario that they believe led to their findings and what, they suspect, will ensue. The article's concluding paragraph summarizes the model and its implications:

If urban prostitutes constitute a major reservoir of AIDS virus in such African capitals as Nairobi, Kigali, and Kinshasa, we may expect that the virus will continue to be spread throughout the African continent by heterosexual men serving as vectors of infection from one community of urban prostitutes to another. Cultural patterns of sexual behavior, along with urban migration of a male work force and attendant disruption of family units, are factors that may facilitate heterosexual transmission of disease in urban centers, with subsequent spread to rural areas. In addition, the relatively high female:male ratio of cases of AIDS in Africa (1:1 in Zaire, compared with 1:16 in the United States), coupled with a high birth rate, raises the possibility that perinatal transmission may result in high rates of the infection among infants and children. To limit the spread of this serious disease in Africa, there is an urgent need to initiate public health education programs directed at modifying sexual behavior and limiting sexual contact with persons in high-risk populations. (Kreiss et al. 1986, 417)

These researchers apparently based this model on their research among prostitutes in the Pumwani estate of Nairobi and the male patients at the Casino STD clinic. They started the research in 1981, a year after the group discovered that over half of a sample of 300 men at Casino who had genital-ulcer disease said that the source of their disease was a prostitute.[5] They began by mapping the location of the bars where the men said they had found the "source" prostitute. *The Lancet* reported on their research in 1983; there was "an apparent geographical clustering of [chancroid] acquisition of infection in the city center and several poorer residential sections" (Plummer et al. 1983, 1294). Based on these findings, they established a research clinic in Pumwani, the "poorer residential section" closest to Casino.

The Canadian and Kenyan team asserted in both the 1983 *Lancet* article and more forcefully in a 1985 article in the journal *Sexually Transmitted Diseases* (D'Costa et al. 1985) that Nairobi's prostitutes are one, "an important reservoir of sexually transmitted disease," and two, "high-frequency transmitters of sexually transmitted disease." In 1983, they suggested that this finding is the main characteristic of the "epidemiology of chancroid and *H. ducreyi* in Nairobi, Kenya" (the title of the article). The main focus of their 1985 article is the "high-frequency transmission" of STDs by prostitutes. I quote at length from the discussion section of the article in order to capture the textual representation of this model:

Sexually transmitted diseases, particularly gonorrhea, are very prevalent among prostitutes in Nairobi. Depending on social strata and number of clients daily, up to 70% of prostitutes have at least one STD. The prevalence of gonococcal infection among women in residential section A [Pumwani] of Nairobi is comparable to that observed by Meheus et al. in Rwanda. Prostitutes may be a major reservoir of PPNG [penicillinase-producing *Neisseria gonorrhoeae*] in Kenya. Since most of these women are very active sexually, they are high-frequency transmitters of STD.

Sexually transmitted diseases have been ranked as the sixth most important health problem in Africa. Many African countries have

no programs for control of STD. The epidemiology of STD in
Africa differs substantially from that in Western nations. Prostitutes are the most important transmitters of STD in Nairobi
(L. J. D'Costa, unpublished data), Ethiopia, and Rwanda. Rapid
modernization, urbanization, political upheaval, and underdeveloped economies have led to a situation where men migrate to cities
without their families to seek employment. This large group of unattached men make up the clientele of prostitutes. Such men, infected by prostitutes, subsequently transmit infections to their
regular sex partners when they visit their [the men's] homes in
rural areas. (Plummer et al. 1985, 67)

The model can be characterized briefly in the following way. We start
with an urban "reservoir" of STDs in Nairobi and the absence of
STD-control programs in Africa. Migrant men pay to have heterosexual
vaginal intercourse with women who, as part of that reservoir, have
STDs and frequent heterosexual sex. Migrant men leave the city with
the STD, have (heterosexual) sex at "home" with their "regular" sexual
partners, thus infecting rural women. The system is fueled by three
nonbiological factors: the migration of "unattached" men from rural areas to the city; the absence of economic opportunity for women who do
not have husbands; and the return migration of men to rural homes. All
three factors result from "rapid modernization, urbanization, political
upheaval, and underdeveloped economies."

I want to note several important features of what I call their high-
frequency transmitter model as it is described in this article and repeated in nearly every subsequent publication from this group. First, the
epidemiological origin of the prostitutes' STDs, the "reservoir," is unspecified. The presence of "astounding" rates of infection among prostitutes is taken as a given; it is not understood as the result of any human actions or relationships. The transmissions of interest are those
that originate in the prostitute's body and move to her male clients;
those that result in the prostitute's infection are not a part of the pic-
ture. Second, given the reservoir, men's risk of getting infected in Nairobi appears to be determined only by whether or not they pay for sex.
The degree of risk seems to be unaffected by any other conditions in
which that sex might take place, such as with or without condoms. The
research team does not take up the issue of safer or protected sex until
after the appearance of HIV. Third, women, both prostitutes and regular sexual partners, are stationary factors in this model. They do not
move. They are also entirely separate groups of women. Men, on the

other hand, are "unattached" and mobile. They are both urban and rural. They are also, it seems, all (African or Kenyan) men or any (African or Kenyan) man, indivisible and everywhere.

It is crucial to note that the high-frequency transmitter model, and the construction of Kenyan prostitutes associated with it, was not plucked by these researchers out of thin air. In Western Europe and the United States, as well as in their Asian and African colonies, women, particularly sex workers, have frequently been described as "vectors" of STDs.[6] The researchers built on a history of scientific writing about women's role in the spread of STDs.

The application of the prostitute-plus-migrating-male scenario to the explanation of apparently high rates of syphilis and gonorrhea in Nairobi and other colonial cities was already evident before World War I. Colonial anxieties about the rising numbers of single women in the cities and about where to locate "native" residents were expressed in debates about venereal-disease control in which European and U.S. scapegoating of prostitutes combined with imperialist notions about African sexuality.

The research conducted on STDs in Nairobi and elsewhere in Africa during the 1960s and 1970s further developed the prostitute-as-reservoir model. For example, during the 1970s, European medical scientists explained the emergence of penicillin-resistant gonorrhea in Nairobi by describing "a 'promiscuous women pool' (PWP) catering for [urban men's] sexual needs" (Verhagen et al. 1971, 278; Verhagen and Gemert 1972; Hopcraft et al. 1973). Similar arguments were made based on research in Kampala, Uganda (Kibukamusoke 1965; Arya and Bennett 1967). The concept of the prostitute reservoir has more recently appeared as a fact that defines the epidemiology of STDs in Africa generally (Holmes 1992; Holmes, Sparling, and Wasserheit 1998).

AIDS has not changed the basic elements of the old model. In their first article on AIDS (Kreiss et al. 1986), Plummer's group uses the high-frequency transmitter model to explain the appearance of AIDS in East Africa and to predict an epidemic of "AIDS virus" infection in the rest of Africa. The following fragments from the conclusions of this article are indicative: "If urban prostitutes constitute a major reservoir of AIDS virus . . . heterosexual men serving as vectors of infection from one community of urban prostitutes . . . urban migration of a male work force and attendant disruption of family units . . . subsequent spread to rural areas" (417). The prostitute reservoir, the mobile male vectors,[7] and the rural victims are all in place.

The model has been modified to respond to some of the new ques-

tions raised by HIV, however. A source of HIV in the prostitutes is acknowledged (or at least "suspected"): "transcontinental spread [by men]
from Central Africa rather than introduction of the virus by visitors
from Europe or North America" (Kreiss et al. 1986, 417). This is an
important change. Before AIDS, there seemed to be no need to explain
how prostitutes were first infected with STDs. The origin of AIDS,
however, was a highly politicized question, the answer to which could
neither be taken for granted nor ignored at the time this article was
written and published. AIDS not only introduced a new question (How
did these prostitutes get infected?), it also seemed to demand a con-
sciousness of national borders and their permeability, at least to men.

Over time, other modifications were made to the high-frequency
transmitter model. The most evident changes appear in the nature and
degree of "difference" specified between Kenya's or Africa's epidemiological pattern and that of European or North American countries. In
the group's first article, the only difference implied lay in the relative
availability of diagnostic technology (Nsanze et al. 1981).[8] With the
arrival of AIDS, however, the difference between Europe and North
America on the one hand and Africa on the other is made both greater
and more epidemiologically significant. The high-frequency transmitter
model is presented as the virtual opposite of that characterizing the
"situation" in, specifically, the United States. Not only is this difference important but it appears to be a main goal of the article to demonstrate that there could be no causal relationship between the epidemic
in the United States and that in Africa. In their first article on AIDS,
the finding that prostitutes whose main clientele were "North Americans or Europeans" were less likely to be infected than those whose
partners were from Rwanda, Burundi, Uganda, or Kenya is deemed crucial; it is reemphasized in the conclusions: "None of the prostitutes in
the low socioeconomic class had had sexual contact with a non-African"
(Kreiss et al. 1986, 417). We have never learned which men gave Nairobi's prostitutes their first non–HIV-related STDs.

Another modification of the model hinted at in this article becomes
quite important in subsequent research and, ultimately, in the development project that emerged out of this research. At the very end of their
1986 article, Kreiss's team takes the effects of high-frequency transmission one step further. From rural sexual partners, the virus may be
transmitted to fetuses or newborns. The pregnant woman, the mother,
and the child have now been added to the model. As we shall see, this
eventually provides a new site of intervention, one which can be made
to fit nicely with the emphasis on AIDS as a development crisis that

emerged at the World Health Organization and other international organizations during the early 1990s.

Just as the model is embedded in multiple histories of moral and medical understandings of STDs, it has also been applied to the spread of HIV by researchers in other countries. In his brief critique of what he calls the "urban disease model," Philip Setel notes that the view of prostitutes as a "core"[9] group of viral transmitters became an influential explanation for the spread of HIV in northern Tanzania (1999, 208–209). Pheterson (1990) also summarizes some of this work and points out just how obsessed with urban sex workers the medical research on HIV in Africa has been. At least in the early years of the epidemic, however, the Nairobi research team's model got the most attention.

The many articles that have come out of the multinational research project are organized according to this basic model.[10] The Plummer group has become best known for its work on how other STDs serve as what they have termed co-factors in the acquisition of HIV. From early in the epidemic, AIDS researchers were puzzled by two consistent findings: one, that not everybody who has unprotected sex with an HIV-antibody–positive person becomes HIV-antibody positive herself; and two, that HIV spreads faster among some people than it does among other people. It is not surprising that the microbiologists sought microbiological explanations for both of these findings. Since they had determined already that prostitutes were reservoirs and high-frequency transmitters of both ulcer-causing STDs and HIV, they hypothesized that perhaps these two infections were linked. They suspected that ulcer-causing STDs made the prostitutes who had them even more "efficient" transmitters of HIV to their migrant male clients. Based on this hypothesis, they narrowed their sights once more on genital ulcers in the Pumwani prostitutes.

The lead story of the August 19, 1989, issue of *The Lancet* presents most clearly the microbiological version of the high-frequency transmitter model. The article is entitled "Female-to-Male Transmission of Human Immunodeficiency Virus Type 1: Risk Factors for Seroconversion in Men" (Cameron et al. 1989). This title must have been a bit startling to the readers of the journal. By this time, HIV researchers had learned that during unprotected vaginal intercourse, women were more likely to get HIV from an infected man than men were to be infected by an HIV-positive woman (Johnson and Laga 1988). Regardless of their intention, the title would have suggested that the authors were offering a departure from what was becoming accepted knowledge about the relationships among biological sex, gender, and HIV.

Like so many others, this article begins by reminding us of the "fundamental regional difference" between HIV epidemiology in Africa and that in "Europe and America" (403). And again the authors suggest that their research provides the explanation for this difference. This time, however, the focus is not on how many prostitutes have HIV or who they will infect. The text emphasizes instead how prostitutes spread HIV to their male clients. The authors follow a certain logic: men infected with an STD and likely to be clients of prostitutes are likely to get HIV. Such men can thus be followed to see how many get HIV and when.[11] The study followed 422 male patients at Casino who reported having had sex with a prostitute and no one else within four weeks of coming to the clinic with an STD. The men in the sample who became HIV positive, concluded the researchers, had gotten HIV from the prostitute at the same time they got the ulcer-causing STD.

But how did the prostitutes infect the men? The team of researchers offer their interpretation of the data in several articles (Cameron et al. 1989; Kreiss et al. 1989; Kreiss et al. 1994; and Plourde et al. 1994). Cameron and his co-authors claim that

> an ulcer raises the infectivity of an HIV-1 infected woman by increasing virus shedding in the female genital tract. This process could be mediated by the recruitment and activation of HIV-1 infected macrophages and lymphocytes to the disrupted epithelial surface by the local inflammatory response, and direct contact of infectious exudate and blood with the genital epithelium of the susceptible [male] sexual partner. (1989, 406)

The microbiological model reiterates the epidemiological model of high-frequency transmission. It again centers on prostitutes and assumes that the first and most important line of transmission is from prostitute to "susceptible" man.

The Nairobi team's research on mothers and babies is also organized according to the high-frequency transmitter model. As the model suggests, the problem of perinatal STD and HIV transmission is of secondary interest.[12] This follows logically from the model in which researchers position infection of mothers and newborns at the geographic and epidemiological periphery, as the eventual outcome of prostitutes' sexual and microbiological behavior and male migration. The articles on mothers and newborns assume that this population is entirely distinct from the group of women identified as prostitutes, despite the reality that the maternity hospital where they conducted their research and the cohort of prostitutes are located in the same neighborhood. The high-frequency transmitter model positions rural wives, steady girlfriends, mothers, and especially babies as the final and most innocent victims of the organization of urban heterosexuality. This construction is evident in the articles dealing with pregnant women,[13] despite the fact that at least some of these are probably "urban" mothers. The focus of these studies is the outcome of maternal infection: babies with low birth weights, dead babies, or babies who will die because their mother is going to die.

The Evidence

Evidence certainly exists to support the arguments made by Plummer and his colleagues at the University of Nairobi. The strongest evidence comes from reports on the levels and timing of HIV infection in different population groups of Kenya. I have no reason to believe that this data is incorrect or even suspect. Unlike many other researchers doing some of the early investigations of AIDS in Africa, the Nairobi group used the best available blood-testing equipment, subjecting blood samples that were initially positive for HIV to a second, more accurate test. Most of their samples were fairly large, reducing the likelihood of error. Moreover, they were able to do a retrospective study of blood samples from the late 1970s up to the early 1980s (Greenblatt et al. 1988). These samples gave them better information on the timing of the epidemic than the simple cross-sectional studies on which most research has been based.

Their retrospective study of frozen blood samples taken from prostitutes and men with chancroid demonstrates that the prevalence of HIV antibody in prostitutes rose from 4 percent in 1981 to 61 percent in 1985. Over the same period, antibody prevalence among men with chancroid went from 0 to 15 percent. No pregnant women sampled had antibodies in 1981 and only 2 percent were infected by 1985 (Piot et al. 1987, 1108). Cross-sectional studies showed the same trends. By 1992, over 80 percent of prostitutes were HIV positive. The rate had risen much more slowly among pregnant women; 13 percent of women in one Nairobi antenatal clinic were infected by 1992 (Plourde et al. 1992, 86). Among all women with an STD, women who were prostitutes were seven times more likely to have HIV than women who had never been prostitutes (86). Based on this data, the argument that HIV spread first and most quickly to prostitutes and then more slowly to men with STDs and that pregnant women were well behind these other groups seems to be a strong one.

The researchers suggest that they derived their model from their data on men's use of prostitutes and wives' reported fidelity, as well as on actual STD and HIV infection among women selling sex. Again, they present data that supports this, although there is no discussion of this data until well after the high-frequency transmitter model is considered to be a fact. In 1994, Moses and his colleagues reported that 37 percent of married men claimed they were infected by a prostitute. By contrast, 74 percent of married women said they had been infected by their husbands (Moses et al. 1994). Based on these reports, it seems that the theory that Nairobi's men, particularly those with STDs, have a lot more sexual intercourse than women, particularly women identified as wives, is a fairly good one.

The more general claims that HIV is concentrated among African prostitutes and that male migration is an important factor in the spread of HIV also find support. There is good evidence from other capital cities in sub-Saharan Africa that sex-worker populations have much higher rates of HIV infection than do women and men who report that they do not exchange sex for money (U.S. Bureau of the Census 2002). Anthropologists lend support to the claim that the circular movement of single men between rural and urban areas influences the extent and shape of the epidemic in sub-Saharan Africa. Rates of HIV seropreva-lence remain higher in Kenya's three largest cities (Nairobi, Mombasa, and Kisumu) than in any of the country's smaller towns and villages (U.S. Bureau of the Census 2002). Janet Bujra and Carolyn Baylies found that in Zambia and Tanzania, large differences in urban and ru-ral rates of HIV infection, and even the existence of AIDS, are ex-plained locally as an effect of rural-to-urban migration (2000, 30). Brooke Grundfest Schoepf (1997) has found that in Zaire, colonial and postcolonial economic pressures have consistently pushed young men out of rural areas and into the cities; she lists this as one of several trends influencing the spread of HIV in that country. Philip Setel (1999) finds similar patterns in Tanzania. A few studies have docu-mented the increases in HIV that have occurred in towns and cities that lie close to common trading routes (Nkya et al. 1991; Bwayo, Omari, et al. 1991; Bwayo, Mutere, et al. 1991; Caldwell and Caldwell 1993). Nai-robi, Mombasa, and Kisumu are all important national, regional, and even subcontinental trading centers. Men are the primary transporters in long-distance trade. Such material supports the North Americans' argument that male mobility is a crucial feature of the epidemiology of HIV in Nairobi.

The group's influential co-factor theory is well supported by their own data. Certainly rates of ulcer-causing STD infection were very high among the prostitutes in Pumwani. In 1985, 71 percent of the women they recruited from this area had at least one of these STDs. Many had two or three. The high rates of HIV they subsequently found among the prostitutes are suggestive of the associations they later studied. Moreover, in 1992, they reported that women with a genital ulcer were between two and five times more likely to have HIV compared to women without an ulcer-causing disease (Plourde et al. 1992). The finding that HIV existed in the discharge from prostitutes' ulcers is also important. The group reported that Pumwani Maternity Hospital experienced "a rapid rise in the prevalence of both HIV-1 infection and syphilis in pregnant women with relatively low-risk sexual behaviour," suggesting that the co-factor theory might hold for the women they believed to be "secondary" cases of HIV (Temmerman et al. 1991, 1181). Finally, the data on men supports the co-factor theory as well. In their prospective study of HIV infection in over 400 men who had STDs, the research team found that men who reported that they had gotten their genital-ulcer disease from a prostitute were the mostly likely to become HIV positive during the period under study (Cameron et al. 1989).

In short, both their own data and that of others suggest that at least some of the things one would expect if the high-frequency transmitter model were a good representation of reality are in fact present in Nairobi, at least among the groups the researchers have defined and studied. Pumwani's prostitutes do seem to have been infected earlier than Casino's men. The men were apparently infected earlier and certainly at higher rates than several samples of pregnant women. If self-reported sexual behavior is to be trusted and if women and men are equally likely to report their actual experiences, then the expectation that men have more sex with more different partners than women do is also borne out by the data. Finally, male migration is likely to be a crucial epidemiological factor.

There is, however, some reason to question just how well the high-frequency transmitter model fits the data collected by the researchers who present it as well as data provided by other researchers. In order to see where the problems lie, it is necessary to look further at the methods that produced the data gathered by the model's authors. The first article to report on the high rates of STDs among Pumwani's prostitutes, and therefore the study that laid the groundwork for developing the claim that these women serve as a "reservoir" for such diseases (Plummer et al. 1983), is problematic. The authors provide a map which they say shows the "probable geographical sources" of the genital-ulcer infections that men at Casino have. The map, they claim, shows the bars in which their male subjects found the prostitutes who then gave those men genital ulcers. The fact that the bars associated with the most infections are located near each other in a particular part of town (which turns out to be Pumwani) is supposed to tell us that there is an "apparent geographical clustering of acquisition of infection in the city center and several poorer residential sections" (Plummer et al. 1983, 1294).

At first glance, this seems an interesting and useful way to study the issue; the mapping of sexual networks and disease transmission has given us a lot of information on the social as well as biological relationships involved in HIV transmission. Oddly, however, the article reports that only 10 percent of the infections among their male patients can be traced to prostitutes working in any of these bars. We are not told from where the other 90 percent came. Nonetheless, we have, it seems, identified the "reservoir." This study marks the beginning of the team's now nearly twenty-year study of the Pumwani prostitutes, on whom their model rests. The initial selection of these women seems to have been based on relatively little evidence, unless it is reasonable to label as a "reservoir" a geographical cluster of women who spread 10 percent of one type of STD identified in a health clinic near that location. Even if 10 percent is a sufficiently high level to constitute a "reservoir," one might wonder what model might have emerged had Plummer and his group studied women and men in other parts of town. It is interesting that the authors themselves comment at the end that "the implications of these data for the design of control programmes are somewhat uncertain, because of the small number of proven female transmitters of *H. ducreyi* studied directly" (Plummer et al. 1983, 1295). Nonetheless, their subsequent articles build upon this same limited data, frequently citing this article as evidence for their model.[14]

There is also the question of how the researchers knew which STDs or HIV infections in Casino's male patients came from Pumwani's prostitutes. The research team relied exclusively on men's own reports of which women had given them a disease. Often, it seems, a woman was presumed to be the source simply if she was a prostitute (again, we do not know how this was determined). Plummer's group explains this method by way of defining what a "source contact" is:

> A woman was considered a source contact if her ulcer symptoms preceded those in the male partner by ≥ 7 days or if she was a prostitute or had had sexual partners other than the male member of the contact pair within the last month and the male partner denied having other sexual partners within the previous month. (Plummer et al. 1983, 1293)

Men's "denial" of having had sex with anyone other than the woman he blames for his infection is accepted as truth. The articles never mention similar discussions with prostitutes about their "source contacts." Nor are prostitutes ever asked to confirm the men's reports.

Are such self-reports reliable? In chapter 2, I noted that several of the staff members at Casino scoffed at the idea that men's stories about how they got infected, who else they might have infected, or whether they use condoms could actually be believed. There was a wide consensus that male patients at Casino were irresponsible and that they often lied to the staff. Even if the staff were overstating this, it does nonetheless make me question the validity of the self-reports and the researchers' apparently unproblematic and unquestioning acceptance of these reports.

The numbers in these articles are at times confusing and even questionable. Dr. L. J. D'Costa, then doctor-in-charge at Casino, provided "unpublished data" that 90 percent of men with gonorrhea got it from prostitutes. This still-unpublished figure did not appear in the medical reports of the clinic, which does not keep written records of where patients say they got a disease. My faith in this data is also weakened by a move that the researchers made between the 1983 publication and a 1985 article. In 1983, they asserted that 57 percent of the men at Casino reported that a prostitute was the source of their genital-ulcer disease (Plummer et al. 1983, 1293). In 1985, the researchers claimed that in the 1983 study they had found that "prostitutes were implicated in the infections of two-thirds of men with genital ulcers" (D'Costa et al. 1985, 64). It is disconcerting at best to see the researchers apparently inflating their own numbers.

There is an even deeper methodological problem in the study. How is it, I asked the texts, that a "prostitute" is defined and identified? Well before the AIDS crisis began, sex workers and feminist scholars had demonstrated that sex work is everywhere a highly complex and internally differentiated category of labor and social experience.[15] Studies of prostitution in sub-Saharan Africa have shown that both single and married women engage in a number of different economic, domestic, romantic, and sexual relationships that involve some kind of payment by a male partner or client. These include temporary monogamous or polygamous marriages, or "town marriages" (Kibukamusoke 1965; Obbo 1980 and 1993; Davis 2000); occasional sexual intercourse offered along with numerous other domestic or productive services (White 1990; Mbilinyi and Kaihula 2000); short-term sexual exchanges between teen-aged women and older wealthy men in return for monetary or other "gifts," often referred to as "sugar daddy" relationships (Doyal 1994; Bujra and Baylies 2000); legalized state-controlled prostitution and the illegal industry such state control usually produces (Renaud 1997); hotel-based encounters, often with foreign men and soldiers (Outwater 1996); and brothel-based prostitution, typically managed by older women who have retired from the business (Tandia 1998). Several studies suggest that women also move among these different types of unions as their needs and health change over their lifetimes (White 1990; Schoepf 1997).

Luise White's in-depth historical research (1990) demonstrates that within Pumwani itself there have been and continue to be many different types of sexual unions and exchanges. White also indicates that women interpret their work and label themselves in a variety of ways; thinking of oneself as and calling oneself a "prostitute" is probably the least common of these (see also Tabet 1989). Studies by other researchers suggest that the definition of a prostitute is important and that medical researchers should consider the question to be unresolved. Pattullo, Masio, and Malisa (1993) reported that among 142 women with genital-ulcer disease at Casino, only "a minority" identified as prostitutes. Twenty-five percent of the women reported "trading sex for goods or money at some time, but did not consider themselves to be prostitutes" (732). Moreover, such trading was not significantly associated with HIV infection.

This diversity does not in itself make the data incorrect. It does, however, suggest the possibility that these researchers, while claiming to be discovering an epidemiological reality, are in fact creating it. Did women in Pumwani come to define themselves as "prostitutes" once they entered the study? Did they ever identify as prostitutes, or is that simply a convenient, long-lived, formulaic homogenizing term applied or transferred from old research? Were all the women who signed up for the study really selling sex for money? Although women risked their reputations by joining a "prostitute" study, enrollment did offer benefits that must have been very attractive to many low-income women. Subjects received access to good-quality, free health care services at the research clinic. Their participation protected them at least somewhat from police harassment (which is often directed at any woman found alone after dark) because Plummer's group was well known and well respected in the area. The women subjects were able to participate in various kinds of discussion and counseling groups.[16] They received condoms whenever they wanted them and were not negatively judged for requesting them.[17] All women should have these things. In Nairobi, however, most do not. In such a context, the incentive to sign up and "play" a prostitute could be significant.

A closely linked problem of identification is the high-frequency transmitter model's suggestion that prostitutes and pregnant women are entirely distinct groups. The persistence and danger of constructions of women as either mother-madonna or prostitute-whore are all too famil-

iar to feminists. A number of researchers have tried to call policymakers' and scientists' attention to the fact that such simplistic binary oppositions allow women who do not define themselves using the categories provided to believe that they are not at risk (Carovano 1991; Setel
1999; Treichler 1999).[18] The Plummer group's assumption that mothers
and whores are distinct and mutually exclusive groups makes pregnancy
and mothering among women who sell sex invisible. Despite rare references to the possibility that some prostitutes have been "abandoned" by
husbands (and therefore have been in relationships that might produce
children even if we assume that paid sex would not), pregnancy is not
referred to in the articles focusing on prostitutes. Although the high
rates of STDs among prostitutes may have made some proportion of
them less fertile and although they are more likely to use contraceptives
than other Kenyan women, it seems unlikely that none of them had
been pregnant, had considered becoming pregnant, or was a mother at
some point during the research.

On the other side, mothers are always assumed not to be selling sex.
If poor and working-class women move from long-term marriages to
temporary marriages to multiple unions and back to longer-term marriages over the course of their lifetimes, then it is likely that at least
some of the women in one group also belong to the other group—or
have belonged to it at another time. Moreover, pregnancy among teen-
aged women is reportedly quite high in Nairobi and in Kenya as a whole
(Odongo and Ojwang 1990). If these women are exchanging sex for cash
or other forms of support from so-called sugar daddies, as seems to be
sometimes the case, where are they in the model? In short, the boundary
between the categories of prostitute and mother are likely to be much
less clear or fixed than the researchers assume.

There is no discussion of mothers' sexual behaviors at all. The focus
of research on women who are not prostitutes is on their "obstetrical
outcomes" (Temmerman et al. 1991). I do not mean to suggest that it is
unreasonable to study what happens to infants who are born to women
with HIV or other STDs. Indeed, the Belgian researchers in the STD
research group have done some very important work in this area. However, the explicit purpose of their articles on mothers is not to discover
how or why the women had gotten infected or who these women might
subsequently infect during heterosexual intercourse. The problem is
that none of the biomedical articles published by this group asks such
seemingly significant questions. According to the logic of the model, the
only important results of infection among pregnant women are sick babies. There are women who are too sexual, who are shedding the virus,
and who are, therefore, dangerous transmitters (Kreiss et al. 1994).

There are women who give birth and are likely to have sick or dead babies—but who apparently should not be considered dangerous, or even sexual, as a result. The lack of information on the mothers' actual sexual behaviors as well as on the prostitutes' reproductive behaviors suggests that the researchers are not testing but are rather assuming their model.[19]

Why is all of this important for understanding the politics and the experience of AIDS in Kenya? In her discussion of how women were (too) slowly written into AIDS discourse in the United States, Paula Treichler (1988a) describes the androcentric biomedical model of the early 1980s. She argues that this model was based on an initial assumption that women were immune to HIV. Subsequently, when heterosexual transmission was "discovered," the contagious prostitute and the mother who threatened to wipe out future generations by passing HIV on to babies were added to the model. Treichler concludes that the resulting paradigm made the processes by which women become infected and women's experiences of the resulting illnesses irrelevant to AIDS research and policymaking. It did, however, allow many women, including those who were at very high risk of becoming infected, to believe that they were not affected by the epidemic. Long after data on women's risks was available, this early model kept in place a belief that HIV/AIDS was and would remain "contained" in apparently isolated communities of gay men, injecting drug users (usually assumed to be male and African-American or Latino), and African sex workers.[20]

Despite the claims of North Americans and Western Europeans that "African AIDS" was totally different from AIDS in their own countries, parts of the androcentric and racist model used in Europe and the United States to explain venereal disease were imported by researchers trying to analyze HIV/AIDS in Africa.[21] The virtual obsession with women who could somehow be identified as prostitutes and the inability to see that such women were probably not part of clearly bounded sexual communities are the effects, in part, of the migration of the Euro-American model. Twenty years after the start of the epidemic and in the face of very high rates of infection in nearly every community, it is still common to assume that AIDS comes from prostitutes, that "good" women will not get infected, and that if such women do become HIV positive either they were prostitutes after all or their men were engaging in risky behaviors with prostitutes. Such assumptions help reinforce the fiction that some people (whoever does not think of herself as a prostitute or as the wife of a man who has ever visited a prostitute) are immune and do not need to change their behaviors, talk about this disease, or join in efforts to improve conditions for people with HIV.

The Metaphors

One very important way in which the Nairobi HIV/STD research project has continued to fuel this perception is through the metaphors the researchers rely on to describe the women in their Pumwani cohort.[22] Medical sociologists and anthropologists have long argued that the metaphors, images, and analogies we use to explain or describe illness experiences express individual and collective anxieties about survival and the security of economic and political systems in which we have a stake. Certain representations of disease and of the diseased become authoritative because they are used by those who have power, because those who make pronouncements on disease are widely perceived as legitimate or expert, or because those who have power are also perceived to be the most legitimate producers of knowledge about illness. Authorized metaphors affect the way we cope with illnesses and how we treat (or neglect) those we perceive to be at risk of the disease. They influence our assessments of whether we are vulnerable to a disease and what we think of ourselves as a result of our apparent vulnerability or immunity.

Although we always and necessarily use metaphors to speak or write about our bodies, some diseases become widely known and discussed through metaphors that have significant social meanings and consequences. Scientific and popular discourses about highly contagious diseases such as tuberculosis, sexual diseases such as syphilis, and diseases that are new, unpredictable, and incurable such as cancer have been especially full of stigmatizing metaphors.[23] Probably no disease, however, has produced an "epidemic of signification" (Treichler 1988b and 1999) as large, as stigmatizing, and as persistent as AIDS has.[24]

Gail Pheterson (1990) has pointed out that scientific and particularly biomedical language has long used negative metaphors to associate prostitutes with disease and to legitimate research and interventions targeting prostitutes. The language used by the Nairobi HIV/STD Project team in its published articles participates in this history. In their publications, prostitutes are rarely referred to simply as women. Prostitutes are repeatedly described collectively as a "reservoir" and as "high-frequency transmitters." These metaphors are both dehumanizing, albeit in different ways. A reservoir is a manmade (and it usually is men) container, or the result of a manmade barrier, that is typically used to collect and hold surplus water or other valuable resources for various human purposes. In the model, this reservoir has gone stagnant. The reservoir continues to quench a thirst but now the drinker pays a great deal more than a few shillings for the drink; he pays, potentially, with his life.

The metaphor of high-frequency transmission also suggests a human creation. It refers to one of the set of machines that has made certain forms of globalization, including the rapid spread of new biomedical information, possible: a high-tech communication machine. The prostitutes are broadcasting HIV and, of course, new data on HIV.

Other metaphors are less obvious but make apparent the construction of prostitutes as culprits in the spread of HIV and STDs. Like criminals, they are "implicated" in the infections of men. Men are never described as "implicated" in the infection of anyone, including their wives or infants. Only the prostitutes are described as "harboring" various sexually transmitted viruses and bacteria; they are, it is implied, providing safe sanctuary for these evil pathogens, which are just waiting to be transmitted to the "susceptible" men.[25]

The discussion of the presence of HIV in the genital ulcers of prostitutes is couched in language that implies that prostitutes are intentionally mobilizing the virus in their vaginas in preparation for transmission. I repeat an earlier quote, emphasizing this time the metaphors at work:

> An ulcer raises the infectivity of an HIV-1 infected woman by increasing *virus shedding* in the female genital tract. This process could be mediated by the *recruitment* and *activation* of HIV-1 infected macrophages and lymphocytes to the disrupted epithelial surface by the local inflammatory response, and direct contact of infectious exudate and blood with the genital epithelium of the susceptible [male] sexual partner. (Cameron et al. 1989, 406; emphasis mine)[26]

The prostitute's body here is not simply a passive reservoir of STDs. Like animals, prostitutes actively "shed" the virus from their genitals. The image of "shedding" suggests both a sloughing off, as if the prostitute can get rid of it from her body like a snake sheds its skin, and a significant and forceful outward flow of the virus, like a dog shedding water. Men and mothers with genital ulcers and HIV are never described as "shedding" a virus. The prostitute's body is not just shedding the virus, moreover. It is recruiting and activating the virus. These words suggest that the body of the prostitute is calling all viral material to her genitals and then preparing it for heterosexual transmission and infection of the male. The man's epithelium (the tissue covering the penis) is merely susceptible; it is the prostitute's victim.[27] This is an especially interesting metaphor, given the multitude of studies that have argued that two important reasons that male-to-female transmission appears to be much more "efficient" than the reverse[28] are one, that the penis more forcefully ejaculates infected fluid than women's genitals do (Zierler 1994), and two, that women's cervixes, particularly when women are young, are more fragile and easily torn than men's genital areas (Ehrhardt 1996).

In short, the purportedly objective high-frequency transmitter model transmits the message that prostitutes cause sexual diseases in men (and their innocent wives and babies). It posits that how prostitutes got infected in the first place is irrelevant; that it is, indeed, a meaningless question. The model justifies a view that as prostitutes, Kenyan women can be experimented on; their vaginas can be and in fact should be probed repeatedly to answer researchers' questions.

The Social Geography: Pumwani

In order to understand how, why, and with what effects the high-frequency transmitter model represents and misrepresents women's sexuality and their responsibility for the spread of HIV, I want to re-insert that model back into the social geography and history of Nairobi from which biomedicine extracts it. Like Harvey, the invisible rabbit in the play of the same name (Chase 1953), the neighborhood of Pumwani is the ever-present but unseen character in the texts produced by the Nairobi research group. Pumwani is the community from which the prostitutes are recruited for the research. It is the location of the prostitutes-only research clinic established by the group. It is where, we are to assume, all the sex and high-frequency transmission that has produced this epidemic happens. It is the residential area closest to Casino, the STD clinic where the research project started.

In the medical articles published by Plummer's multinational team of researchers, however, Pumwani's presence and organization are taken for granted. Aside from one or two comments in the early papers that Pumwani is "notorious" for prostitution and one of a number of "poorer residential sections" of the city, Pumwani is just a name—now somewhat famous, as in "the Pumwani cohort" that various articles refer to—but only a name, nonetheless.

Pumwani's history is very important, however, to the explanation of how this research came about and why it has taken the form of a model blaming prostitutes. Pumwani's history as part of the larger story of European imperialism in Kenya has made the neighborhood an ideal site for such research. The area was originally called Pangani. It was settled by Africans who were, by definition, squatting illegally in the city reserved for whites. After World War II, Pangani was razed by colonial officials, who created in its place a more permanent and controllable neighborhood called Pumwani.

Located near the city's major markets and business district, Pumwani was the object of Europeans' anxieties about what they perceived to be the biological, sexual, and political threats posed by urbanizing Africans. Pumwani was settled by women who migrated from the nearby hinterland, sold sexual and other domestic services to employed male migrants, and accumulated sufficient capital to build permanent dwellings (White 1990). In large part because these women and their tenants were already established there, the colonial government defined the neighborhood officially as the city's "African Location." As Luise White convincingly argues in her history of the area, it was Pumwani's groups of part-time and full-time, home-based, street-based, and bar-based sex workers who founded and defined African Nairobi.[29]

Pumwani's sexual and economic geography did much more for the research project than make the neighborhood a convenient place to set up shop. In a country where prostitution is illegal, where the government pretends that there is no sex trade, and where there have been no apparent efforts to organize sex workers into a political constituency, it might be quite difficult to identify a sufficiently large sample of sexually active women and to keep them as a long-term cohort. Moreover, the illegality of prostitution makes the women who practice it vulnerable to the police and allows them little access to public services such as health care (Alexander 1996). Such conditions, combined with the history of close-knit community support among sex workers in Pumwani, have created a large and relatively stable population well suited to STD and HIV research that is based on the assumption that such diseases originate in prostitutes' bodies.

This is never discussed in the articles. As scientific researchers, apparently, we do not need to know that Pumwani has been a site of negotiation and struggle between prostitutes and the state, between colonized Kenyans and colonizing Europeans, and between single Kenyan women and working-class men. We do not need to learn that the women living and working there are the successors of women who chose to exchange their sexual services to construct an urban home for themselves and for men. If we did know all of this, we might begin to question constructions we would otherwise accept or not even notice. We might begin to think about the "Pumwani cohort" as a collection of individual people rather than as high-frequency transmitters. We might wonder how the history of the colonial state and the colonial and postcolonial economies affected these women's risks of getting STDs and eventually

HIV. We might, finally, wonder if the repeated probes into the prostitutes' bodies can really be justified.[30]

Finally, we turn to the politics of heterosexual masculinity—or, rather, the politics of making heterosexual masculinity disappear—expressed in the high-frequency transmitter model. In the biomedical narratives told by Plummer's research team, Kenyan men serve as bridges between the two groups of women, prostitutes and wives or mothers. This bridge, however epidemiologically significant, is very hard to see; it is obscured by the crowds of prostitutes and their shedding genitalia. The behaviors of Kenyan (or any other) men as a group or as individuals are not discussed beyond mention of the men's reports regarding their use of prostitutes. Male research subjects are not grouped according to any actual or assumed sexual behavior or identity; they are merely "patients presenting with an STD." There is no cohort of male clients or husbands/fathers followed over many years. There is no single sample of penises that are repeatedly visited, viewed, and described by researchers. The male samples are drawn from whoever happens to come to Casino for treatment during a specified period. The one prospective study on men required only a few return visits and ended after about sixteen months. We learn nothing from these narratives about the men's class positions or incomes, occupations, residence, or, astonishingly, condom use.

The relative invisibility of men should seem odd. According to the model, the men of Nairobi are the country's movers, the active ones who carry the virus from urban to rural areas, from prostitute to wife, mother, and baby. Without them it would seem that HIV would simply stay contained in the reservoir. I have argued elsewhere that this silence can be read as a probably unconscious unwillingness on the part of researchers, development agencies that fund them, and the state to challenge male sexual power in Kenya or elsewhere (Booth 1995).[31] A more pragmatic conclusion is that as "high-frequency" users of public health services, women are literally more captive research objects than men. These are not mutually exclusive explanations for the absence of men. It is, of course, impossible to establish the authors' or publishers' "true" intentions or meanings. It is only possible and relevant to consider the various effects this discourse is likely to have on readers, including policymakers and other scientists. The silence about masculinity and male sexuality makes it very difficult to imagine interventions that might effectively target Kenyan men individually or, more significant for making long-term change, to address either the assumption or the reality that men will have a great deal of unprotected sex with many different partners.

The most recent research conducted by Plummer's team brings us full circle. After having done so much research on the Pumwani sex workers, and after claiming with some justification to have done so much for the sex workers, the team has started to ask the prostitutes to give the world something of potentially enormous value: an HIV vaccine. In the middle 1990s, Plummer's colleagues announced their discovery that a small group of the prostitutes had never gotten infected with HIV. These women were apparently having as much vaginal intercourse without a condom and with the same men as the women who had gotten infected (Martin et al. 1994; Fowke et al. 1996). A few years after making this discovery, the researchers advanced the hypothesis that the uninfected prostitutes had a genetic distinction that gave them immunity and that this genetic material could be isolated and made the basis for a vaccine (Kaul et al. 2000; MacDonald et al. 2000).

This was exciting news that deserved attention and support, which it has gotten (Vick 2001). In the end, a vaccine might be the only way to stop AIDS. To broadcast the work and mobilize support, Plummer and his colleagues starred in a documentary film called *Searching for Hawa's Secret* (Krotz 1999). The film introduces us to "Hawa," an uninfected Kenyan prostitute, celebrates the team's work so far, and indirectly asks for financial contributions. In the film, Frank Plummer comments that the expense involved in developing a vaccine will exceed at least the short-run profits; pharmaceutical companies are not, therefore, funding projects such as his.[32] He does not say that pharmaceutical companies are also noting that the main market for a vaccine will be the world's poorest people, a reality that is unlikely to increase the interest of such corporations.[33]

The film does not discuss the implications of the research for Hawa and her community except to say that the profits (which promise to be small) from the vaccine, if successful, will be shared in some unstated way with the women in Pumwani. I read the film's title as a no–doubt-unwitting comment on the relationship between the researchers and the sex workers. *Hawa* in Kiswahili means lust, passion, or passionate desire. It is also the Kiswahili name for the biblical Eve. In addition, *hawa* is the demonstrative pronoun "these"—an unnamed collectivity of which the speaker is not a part. At least to those who understand Kiswahili, *Hawa* stands as a symbol for all of these lustful, fallen (even evil) women who might, nevertheless, be rehabilitated by their contribution to modern science.

"These" women have a "secret," however. The North American and European researchers' responsibility is to search for and uncover their secret, which, it is possible to conclude, the sex workers are deliberately hiding. Scenes of Pumwani and references to it as a "slum" make way for scenes of a sterile Canadian laboratory and a large complicated-looking machine that apparently spins Hawa's blood to separate it into different components. But how, ultimately, will Hawa and the other sex workers, whether HIV negative, HIV positive, living with AIDS, or already dead, benefit from this research?

In the film Hawa herself makes a comment that she is proud to have contributed to such important research. Certainly the film does give the sex workers some very sympathetic visibility; it allows viewers to see their humanity in ways that thankfully contrast with all the sensationalist press about infected African whores. It also makes the quite important point that Hawa's infected colleagues are unlikely ever to get good drug treatment for their illnesses, challenging the international community's focus on developing expensive drugs rather than vaccines.

The film does not address several crucial questions, however. On whom will new vaccines be tested first? If a control group is used, will they be told to have risky sex like those whose bodies will be testing the vaccine? If a safe and effective vaccine is ever produced, who will be vaccinated and when? How will a vaccine be made affordable to Kenyan women and men? These questions, of course, can be asked of research on any vaccine and using any sample of people. But the enormous social and economic distance between the now geographically intimate agents of global medical science and local working-class Kenyan women makes the answers much more difficult. It is not only ironic that, having remedicalized and thus relegitimized the blaming of urban African women for spreading sexual disease to male workers, wives, and babies, *Wazungu* researchers are now trying to turn the blood of these women into something which may protect all these others from the same disease. It should also give us pause and make us wonder rhetorically what happens after Hawa has given us all of this. Will a vaccine protect young working-class women from the violence that sex workers experience at the hands of clients and police? Will it allow them to charge enough money for their services to live adequately or, if they wish, to leave sex work for a different, well-paying, safer, and more permanent job?

The work done during nearly twenty years of biomedical research on STDs and HIV/AIDS among heterosexuals in Nairobi silences the historical and current relationships of power on which its production depends. This silencing helps to make the researchers' scientific texts authoritative and influential; in short, it makes them into successful narratives. The story they tell is very appealing. Much of it fits the data. Much of it seems, and probably is, useful to know. Much of it fits the ideas of Africa, of prostitutes, and of HIV to which the narrative's audiences (state policymakers, other scientists, the WHO, CIDA) are already drawn. It does not invite us to see either the past or the present of colonial relations, which are now taking the form of biomedical discovery and the health care sector development project that we encounter in the next chapter. They do not challenge the members of those audiences to think about masculinity—which would be so much harder to address, given the structures of government in Kenya as well as the organization of power within biomedicine.[34]

Can biomedicine, or normal science more generally, be re-engineered in such a way that it can be liberatory? Can it ever contribute to ending the sexual, gender, class, and race inequalities that support the spread of HIV? Stephen Epstein (1996) has argued that AIDS activists in the United States have changed science by appropriating it to justify their demands for faster approval of AIDS drugs, more money for research, better clinical trials, and so on. Some scientists have had to respond to the new challenges to their authority and to their claims of objectivity. Donna Haraway (1988 and 1989) has told feminists that we cannot afford to give up normal science because it is a powerful tool, not just because it is wielded by the powerful and can empower those who become capable of wielding it but also because it has a great deal of explanatory value. In the two clinics where I talked with nurses and where the Nairobi research team worked, however, the patients-cum-research subjects were not mobilized (or, perhaps, motivated) to present the kind of collective and pragmatic challenge that a renegotiation of the language or outcomes of the scientific research would require. Nevertheless, as we shall see in the next chapter, challenges were made and negotiations over the practice of science, however unconscious, small, and difficult to see, did happen. It remains to be seen what the larger, longer-term possibilities for a liberatory AIDS science might be.

Five

"A Husband Can Have a Thousand Girlfriends!"

From Casino, the downtown clinic for sexually transmitted diseases (STDs), it is a long, crowded, and very bumpy bus ride to the sprawling "estates," as they are euphemistically called, that house most of the millions of Kenyans who have migrated to the capital since independence. I shifted my fieldwork to a clinic located in one of these periurban estates in order to track the progress of the multinational research team's HIV/STD prevention project. As the virus spread, so did the researchers. With the realization in the late 1980s that HIV was not staying within the boundaries of the "risk groups" that had already been identified, research and policy interests turned toward the most visible and, to many, the most disturbing effect of this spread: the infection of babies. This shift was accompanied by AIDS experts' new focus on making STD- and HIV-prevention counseling part of maternal and child health care services.

Bestlands Health Centre is a concrete U-shaped building perched on the edge of the Bestlands "site and service estate." Bestlands was among the many former squatter communities razed, rebuilt by the state, and officially annexed to Kenya's capital city between 1970 and 1985. The Nairobi City Commission built the health center in 1981, just before Moi's government was hit by an economic crisis and an attempted coup. The health center's purpose is to provide primary health care services to the ethnically mixed, mostly blue-collar and informal-sector workers who settled there after the squatters' residences had been bulldozed and relocated to land still farther from the city. Although overcrowded, Bestlands is not among Nairobi's poorest estates. Most of the houses are cement, and there is running water in a large number of them. Bestlands boasts a thriving informal economy that employs many of the residents. Both anecdotes and a perusal of patient cards suggest, however, that many factory workers and low-level white-collar workers, including secretaries, clerks, nurses, and teachers, also live in Bestlands and use its health center. Many of the women patients who list their occupation as "housewife" are, according to Bestlands' nurses, temporary migrants from nearby rural areas who have come to the settlement to visit their urban husbands.

The health center sat just a two-minute walk from the estate's single and extremely busy set of benches and market stalls marking the stop for the public buses that link the estate to downtown (a nearly 45-minute trip) and to the industrial area (which is even farther away). Although it was close to the bus stop, I could not see the health center from my seat on the crowded bus. I knew to get off the bus when I saw the yellow-and-orange–striped tent covering the evangelical Christian group that "squatted" without a church building just in front of the health center. Members of this religious group came to Bestlands Health Centre every morning around 7:30 A.M., half an hour before the health center opened. They preached in at least three languages to the standing-room-only crowd of women and children waiting on the open-air porch for prenatal, family-planning, and well-baby services. Squeezed among "the mothers," as Bestlands' nurses called them, I sat, waited, and listened with half an ear to unsolicited biblical exegeses that seemed to deal mainly with the end of the world and how to prepare for it.

At this period in Kenya's history, when things on both political and economic fronts seemed pretty dismal and a horrible virus was taking more and more lives every day, patients might not have thought the prophets off the mark. Charismatic movements and churches were actually becoming more popular and visible in the city at the time. Although they were indifferent to the preachers' presence, the nurses expressed a sense of doom and a hope for the virtually miraculous. All over the country, health centers such as Bestlands had been extremely hard hit by the one-two punch of economic and epidemiological crises during the late 1980s and early 1990s.

The national-level crises were reflected in such extreme scarcity at Bestlands that nurses spent much of their time ripping up books and papers to use as registration cards. The center, which was visited by well over 150 patients on an average day, had only one working sterilizer (which frequently broke down) and two examination tables. The center is designed to have three clinical officers. During the time of my study there was only one, and she was frequently called away to meetings or for trainings. This meant that the nurses often had to perform diagnostic activities for which they were not trained.

The nurse in charge of stocking and handing out drugs, needles, and syringes said to me: "Since there are no medicines and no syringes, sick ones don't come."[1] Bestlands' nurses had been getting fewer packages of drugs, gloves, antiseptic lotion, sterile gauze, and syringes from the government since about 1990. In that year, the government—under the influence of the World Bank—suddenly started requiring patients to pay a portion of the cost of being treated in the country's previously free public clinics. Although the policy failed, the government did not resume its responsibility for buying supplies or drugs.[2] The nurses never knew when the few supplies they might get would show up. Fewer and fewer patients with treatable diseases came to the health center. On occasion, the section of the center devoted to treating acute illnesses, known as the "curative side," would be unexpectedly crowded when I arrived in the morning. These crowds, I learned, were the result of the spread of rumors, sometimes true and sometimes not, that "drugs had arrived" at the health center. People would show up hoping to get whatever was available. Twice during the three months I was there the rumor was true, but both times the drugs ran out before everybody could be treated. More often the rumors were unfounded. Disappointed patients went home to find money to get treated in private clinics or just to suffer a bit longer. The "curative side" of Bestlands therefore saw little action, aside from the patients who came for the project's STD services.

The larger portion of the clinic, that part devoted to preventive health, however, continued to do a relatively good business. This was the product of two factors. First, Kenya's primary health care system was in practice and not coincidentally heavily oriented toward delivering the two kinds of services that donors were interested in funding: family planning and well-baby care, mainly immunizations and advice on nutrition. Although its dispensary rarely had antibiotics, the cupboards on what nurses referred to as the "preventive side" were well stocked with donor-subsidized birth control pills, injectable contraceptives, condoms, intrauterine devices, basic immunizations, and child-survival cards on which mothers were supposed to record their babies' progress. The second reason for the continuing flow of patients to Bestlands' preventive side was its frequent use by the University of Nairobi's nursing school as a place to teach the family-planning section of their courses. Whenever the teachers came with students, they brought specula, gloves, and antiseptic lotion as well as more contraceptives. The extra supplies not only kept the family-planning services going but also allowed Bestlands' staff to do more safely the prenatal exams they otherwise skipped or performed without gloves or sterile equipment.

Despite these relatively favorable conditions, the nurses on the preventive side were often unable to provide even the basic maternal and child health care services. The nurses usually could not offer women intrauterine devices because when the training programs finished, the center did not have enough of the gloves or antiseptic lotion needed to perform the insertions. The center had plenty of condoms but was out of the spermicide the nurses were supposed to give women who took condoms. More seriously, the staff frequently could not do the initial speculum exams of pregnant patients upon which nurses are to make decisions about how (and in what facility) women's pregnancies should be treated. They frequently could not tell a woman if she could expect a difficult or easy pregnancy or if she had any serious infections or internal structural problems that might affect the pregnancy or delivery. As the head family-planning nurse, Grace, told me on my first day at the center: "We have no facilities: no gloves, no lotions [sterilizing soap]. Otherwise we could be doing speculum exams. We cannot do them without lotions or gloves."[3]

As a result of what Bestlands could and could not effectively provide for the people living near it, between 80 and 95 percent of the patients seen by the staff there were women coming in for prenatal, well-baby, and family-planning services. Given that family planning in Kenya is virtually entirely aimed at women and that women are considered to be totally responsible for the health of their children, the relative availability of such services and the scarcity of everything else ensured that men by and large stayed away.

Although the scarcity of drugs frustrated the nurses, the absence of men did not seem to bother them terribly. According to the nurses, women felt free to talk about their reproductive needs and their relationship problems at Bestlands. Grace told me: "The women trust us here. This is a clinic for women."[4] The few men who did come for treatment, whether for STDs or something else, were typically treated unsympathetically. Men entered the clinic from the back and waited standing up in one corner, while seated and wandering women filled the waiting area and the halls. The men's bathroom had been broken for years. The two nurses in charge of STD treatment and counseling at Bestlands, like the nurses at Casino clinic, often spoke very harshly to men for getting STDs and endangering their wives and unborn babies.

As a physical place, Bestlands symbolizes post-independence urban "development" policy just as Casino reflects colonial planning and ideology. Casino's geographic location is a product of colonial anxieties about race and sexuality. Bestlands—the community as well as the center—marks the geography of postcolonial class inequality. Although ostensibly planned and maintained by the state, the area sprawls, merging at its invisible boundaries with similar estates on the ever-growing urban periphery. Bestlands Estate originated in the enormous demand for housing created by poor migrants in the 1960s and 1970s. The city added new sections, called phases, in the 1990s; despite high rates of urban unemployment, rural to urban migration continues to be a common response to landlessness and other manifestations of economic crisis. The frequent and overcrowded buses bringing its residents home from downtown or from the industrial area attest to the reality that opportunities to make a living in rural areas have declined for many Kenyans. They come to the city, find or make their own housing in the peripheral estates, and try to survive in a place of very high formal-sector unemployment and relatively few public services.

The activities and conversations that take place inside Bestlands' health center and inside the Casino clinic expose the difference between Kenya's post-independence health care policy and health care policies under the colonial government. Bestlands Health Centre and its 173 counterparts around the country are supposed to treat all the basic health care needs of the majority of Kenya's population along the lines proposed by the United Nations in 1978. The "health for all" strategy emphasizes redistributing health care to the poor and away from expensive hospital care for the rich (WHO 1978). In addition, Bestlands Health Centre's focus on family-planning services reflects the post-independence interests of donors in, or, perhaps more accurately, their obsession with, population control (Hartmann 1995). In contrast, Casino's services reflect the pre-independence focus on keeping urban African men fit to work for Europeans by targeting what the latter saw as those men's major debilitating diseases (Beck 1981; Curtin 1992, 1998). They also mark the colonizers' virtual indifference to the wide range and interconnectedness of infectious diseases experienced by Kenyans in part as an effect of imperial contact.

The two clinics that anchor this book in the "local" also have several things in common, however. First, they both originated in the desire of vulnerable regimes—that is, the old, post–Mau Mau colonial state and the young, inexperienced, and incompletely legitimated independent state—to mobilize popular support by providing the masses with limited but free social services. Second, by the mid-1980s, when AIDS arrived in Nairobi, both clinics had begun to be abandoned by the state. Finally, despite their different orientations, these two clinics have been equally hard hit by HIV/AIDS. They have also been equally affected by the global and local forces defining AIDS as a development problem.

Bestlands Health Centre is one of five health centers in Nairobi and nearby towns that Frank Plummer's multinational HIV/STD team at the University of Nairobi chose as demonstration sites for their attempt to integrate STD services into general primary health care services, particularly maternal and child health care and family-planning programs.[5] The project's first and most important aim was to address the problem of perinatal HIV transmission by identifying pregnant women who had co-factors for HIV transmission—that is, untreated STDs. They hoped to cure such women and counsel them. In addition, they expected to identify, treat, and counsel the heterosexual partners of the women. They also wanted to train a group of health care workers to do all of this work. The ultimate hope was that the project, once made into policy and carried out at all primary health care centers, would reduce the spread of HIV by identifying sexually transmitted infections before they became ulcers that facilitated HIV transmission. In addition, the policy would reduce the number of patients who sought care at Casino and allow Casino to be turned into a referral clinic for people with more-advanced-stage STDs and people with HIV/AIDS (CIDA 1990).

The STD intervention was a predominantly women-operated and women-utilized program, by default as well as by design. Because the program was introduced in a facility that was organized around the delivery of reproductive and (limited) curative services to mothers and children, it is hardly surprising that its objects were virtually entirely female. The two nurses who dispensed the STD drugs and counseled the patients with STDs were women, as were the clinical officer and the family-planning nurse who conducted many of the initial examinations of patients sent to the project.[6]

Two stories that nurses told me about the early period of the project at Bestlands are indicative, I think, of the misfit of project goals, the crisis-ridden Kenyan state, and the daily operation of the center. The first major problem had to do with drugs. The STD project brought to the center's dispensary a large supply of comparatively expensive drugs at a time when the dispensary's store had dwindled to consist of a stock of aspirin, cough syrup, bandages, and an antibacterial salve. The project was initially planned to be "integrated" with all of the center's services; exams for STDs were to happen at the same time and in the same room as routine prenatal and family-planning exams. The STD drugs supplied by the Canadian International Development Agency (CIDA) were to be distributed from the dispensary where all other drugs (when there were any) were given out. Within a few weeks, however, the staff insisted that the STD project be moved to its own room. Susan, the dispensary nurse, told me:

> Initially we gave drugs with the other patients but it couldn't work because the patients stand at the window [of the dispensary] and stand there swallowing the [STD] drugs when others are standing behind and there are no other drugs [for problems other than STDs]. They saw that other patients were getting drugs and they wanted to know why they weren't. When we get more *dawa* [medicine] we'll go back [to the dispensary] for ordinary patients; we'll definitely move back. So we decided to move the patients into this room [the STD room] and we can even do exams here. We can give condoms, counseling here; otherwise [i.e., back in the dispensary] we couldn't do that.[7]

Some non-STD patients would ask specifically for the antibiotics they saw the STD patients getting; they too wanted to be cured or, perhaps, to take the drug home to a sick child. But the nurses had to say no, the drugs are only for STDs. This got to be too hard for them, so they moved the entire STD project, drugs, staff, examination table, and records into one room, far away from and invisible to patients on the "preventive side." The only part of the project that remained "integrated" was the blood testing; the laboratory nurse continued to run the syphilis tests as well as the few other tests the center was able to do.

The second example of tensions at Bestlands concerned staff training. Mary and Wamuuchi were the first of what were eventually to be many nurses trained by and for the project. Wamuuchi called the training the "AIDS Seminar" and proudly showed me her certificate of completion and the pictures she took during the course. This first training was held in Mombasa at a hotel. The staff were put up at the hotel, paid a small amount of money so they could get food, trained by the Canadian and Kenyan staff of Plummer's research team, and, according to Mary, shown a wonderful time. The project leaders' plan was that after this first training—which was provided to two or three nurses, matrons, or clinical officers from each of the demonstration sites—the staff who had been trained would then train other staff members in a less-informal and less-expensive way. Unfortunately, none of the staff, at least at Bestlands, were interested in getting trained in this way. Mary told me that this was because if they were going to do a training, they too wanted to go to Mombasa, stay in a hotel, and get a per diem allowance.

The nurses' desire to go to Mombasa for a training did not stem from selfishness. Like many civil servants considered to be of little importance, health care workers in Kenya's public clinics are terribly underpaid and, what seemed to be worse, given very little respect. Many of the nurses at Casino and, to a lesser extent, at Bestlands, were quite bitter about how the Ministry of Health and the Nairobi City Commission treated them. I was told many stories about nurses being informed one day that the next day they would start working at a different clinic, located perhaps very far from where they lived or in a place they could not get to by public transportation. Nurses seemed to have no influence over such decisions and were usually given almost no warning. Other nurses had been assigned to carry out activities for which they were not trained. Moreover, all of the nurses were working daily under frustrating conditions of resource scarcity and enormous human need. A desire to get out of town on a paid leave and to receive some respectful attention from "the Europeans" along with a training that most of them told me they did indeed want to have was understandable.

These two problems tell a story all too familiar to critics of development who have observed various well-meaning and well-funded projects in action. Local scarcity—of material resources, of prestige, and of income—often redefines interventions from the perspective of their intended beneficiaries (or of those who, for whatever reasons, are not included in the intervention). In contexts where there is no other source of support, resources intended merely to make a project possible become as important or more important than reaching the actual goals of the project. Government health care spending had shrunk from nearly 8 percent of the total government budget in 1972 to 5.4 percent in 1990 (Turshen 1999, 14) and was continuing to decline. When I was at Bestlands, the effects of this decline had already trickled down to the clinical level, leaving nurses and patients alike desperate for resources. Understandably, the situation worsens when economic crisis and government withdrawal from spending on social services are accompanied by the rapid spread of a new and deadly disease.

This context produced a third local crisis for the project. This one was also about drugs. In their contract with the Minister of Health, CIDA and the University of Manitoba agreed to supply drugs for the project clinics for the first year. By 1991, the Ministry of Health would take over supplying drugs. 1991 came and went. 1992 passed. The research team was still buying drugs for the clinics. One of the consultants working with the project described this dilemma to me in an e-mail message responding to my criticism that the project could not be sustained if and when the researchers left Kenya or ran out of money.

Should [the co-director] have stopped the project due to the GoK [Government of Kenya] reneging on its agreement? I don't know. He's an optimist. He kept supplying drugs while investigating every other route available—World Bank, Bamako Initiative,[8] community pharmacies, user fees, hassling Nairobi and Nakuru [the town with another decentralization project] officials, having STD drugs included in the essential drug kits, etc., etc. He didn't sit on his butt dispensing drugs with largesse. . . . It was never CIDA's intent to supply drugs and other materials. They probably wouldn't have funded that because it would have been patently unsustainable right from the start.[9]

Clearly, the project could not operate without the drugs; the ability to treat quickly and effectively the very real and often quite painful symptoms of STDs made the counseling and partner identification possible. The future of the project was uncertain, however. Kenya was in the middle of a national economic crisis. Foreign advisors and domestic elites alike were calling for reductions in government spending on health care and other social services. The priorities of the ruling party, facing as it was at this time a serious political crisis, did not include providing basic health care or confronting the AIDS crisis. In this context, a drug-centered and therefore expensive project seemed unlikely to get past the demonstration stage.

Bestlands' nurses were very conscious of the importance of the drugs and of the fact that without the project their clinic would be doing very little for the community. Wamuuchi, Mary, and Sister Kiroro quite frequently expressed to me their gratitude to the project for supplying the drugs:

You see we are lucky. [Our center] was chosen for research, so we have research from time to time. It [the initial baseline research for the project] was here in Room 4 [the syphilis-screening room]: HIV, syphilis, gonorrhea, trichomonas, candida. It was [the Department of] Community Health jointly being done with Canadians; the University of Manitoba, is it? They are very generous.[10]

The nurses were also well aware of the fact that having the drugs depended upon the continued interest of the researchers in gathering data. As Mary pointed out: "[The researchers] will leave when they get the information they want," and with them would go the drugs. It is in this context of scarcity and drug dependence, and the local, national, and global forces that produced it, that nurses articulated their perspectives on heterosexuality, masculinity, and the logic of using biomedicine and women's bodies to stop an epidemic.

As I argued in the last chapter, the researchers responsible for implementing the CIDA project at Bestlands came armed with a specific model of "African" heterosexuality. In their high-frequency transmitter model, women (as prostitutes) were the origin and main epidemiological and microbiological culprits in HIV transmission. Men were not the researchers' main concern. In fact, men were virtually invisible in the majority of their publications. Although men might be culpable as carriers in the spread of HIV from high-risk to low-risk populations of women, they were, according to the research reports and to the policies influenced by those reports, unavailable or irrelevant as targets for direct intervention.

The nurses at Bestlands did not reject this model. Although few men came on their own to Bestlands' STD project, when they did, Mary and Wamuuchi assumed that they had been infected by a prostitute, regardless of the men's own stories. After treating one man, Wamuuchi turned to me with disgust in her voice and on her face. As the man sat waiting to be excused from the room, she told me in English:

> This one [the male patient], the wife passed away five years ago, so he went to celebrate. He took beer and went to a prostitute. He did not even know her, when he got the signs. He does not know about AIDS so we have told him about AIDS but he's not hearing properly. We told him to come after one week but the partner, he cannot bring her because he doesn't even know her.[11]

Wamuuchi does not dismiss the patient's culpability; none of us was meant to feel sorry for him. But she and the other nurses did dismiss the possibility that he might change his behavior. They did not suggest that he stop visiting prostitutes, that he bring any of his lovers to the clinic to be examined and treated, or even that he use a condom. In such moments, the nurses seemed to share with the researchers key assumptions about the relationship between gender and heterosexual HIV transmission and about the essential irrelevance of men to efforts to stop AIDS.

The nurses at both Casino and Bestlands, however, were very interested in discussing male heterosexual behavior with me, each other, and their female patients. Unlike the language of medical reports about high-frequency transmitters, the nurses' discussions revolved primarily around "African" men's moral culpability and its implications for biomedical interventions in women's sexuality. At Casino, the construction of male STD patients as sexually irresponsible helped to organize the delivery of health care services there. It was also an almost-constant topic of conversation. A similar view of male sexual and health-seeking behavior permeated the culture of Bestlands.

There were some noticeable differences between the tone of discussions about men at Casino and that of those at Bestlands. At Casino, where men were often seen as patients and where a significant number of the staff were men, the conversations about men's behavior often were done in a humorous tone or exhibited minor frustration or intolerance; the staff seemed to have a tolerant, or perhaps resigned, "boys will be boys" sort of attitude. At Bestlands, by contrast, nurses were frequently quite angry at the usually absent men whose wives, partners, or girlfriends the nurses were treating. This was in large part due, I suspect, to the fact that Bestlands catered mainly to pregnant women, women with young children, and women in need of family planning and that all but three of the nine-member staff were women.

Two quotes from some of the conversations I had with nurses at Bestlands are especially indicative of their negative view of men and masculinity. In one conversation, Sister Kiroro made it clear that her women patients risk serious physical abuse if they try to get their husbands to come for STD treatment: "In fact, you treat them, you tell them to ask their partner [to come], and they tell you they will get a beating." Wamuuchi translated a female patient's story this way: "She says she is faithful to her husband. He works with trailers [trucks]—moves from place to place. She has four kids. She says she is faithful; she didn't even know what happened. I asked her what precautions she takes. She tells me she does not move [have sex] with anybody else except her husband. He moves out [has extramarital sex]. He'll eventually bring her AIDS."[12] These comments suggest that attempts to treat STDs expose the degree to which heterosexuality is an enormously, even dangerously, unequal relationship. Nurses implied that heterosexual marriage renders women sexually powerless. According to the nurses, married women patients are helpless against a masculine sexuality that cannot be restrained even by the threat of disease, however potentially fatal.

While I was not surprised by the nurses' perception of "African women" as men's sexual victims, I was not prepared for the way the nurses presented the problem as an essentially "African" problem; not, that is, a problem that is universal, Kenyan, particular to people of the Luo ethnic group or the Kikuyu ethnic group,[13] found only in the working class, or limited to Nairobi. They assumed, it appeared, that *Wazungu* (European or white) men and, by extension, *Wazungu* women like myself, were fundamentally, inherently different and superior hetero-sexuals.

The nurses emphasized the "problem" of masculine heterosexuality by contrasting it with what they perceived to be "European" behaviors and expectations. According to the nurses, while white men's sexuality can be controlled, because they are white men, "African" men are sexually out of control. As Mary said to me during an STD-treatment session with a woman patient who had syphilis, "This woman has been faithful and now she thinks about AIDS—that's why she is crying." Sister Kiroro continued, "For you Europeans it is easy. You can say he went out with another woman and got a disease. But here, even if you say he is *sick*, you can be thrown out. It's a joke in the African context."[14] These comments were not made to patients; the nurses directed them at me, in English, although often a patient, who very likely could understand us, was in the room.

I cannot know whether this was a performance, conscious or not, for my benefit. Was it something that they did not believe but that they thought I did believe and that I wanted to hear? I did challenge them often. I told them (true) stories about *Wazungu* men who refused to wear condoms, who believed themselves entitled to "move around" (a Kenyan English term for "sleep around"), and who infected their wives, girlfriends, and boyfriends as a result. The nurses listened and some-times nodded at the similarity of our experiences. But they continued to talk about African and *Wazungu* men as (hetero)sexually distinct groups. This does not, of course, prove that the construction was other than a performance for me. It does, I think, suggest that the construction was at least relatively comfortable, accessible, and rugged. In any case, I am interested less in discovering the nurses' "authentic" beliefs than in describing and explaining the discourse of the health care center as a negotiation among *Wazungu* researchers, including myself, bio-medicine, nurses, and patients.

The nurses' accounts of female patients' situations told me another story as well: a story about how the nurses perceived themselves. In addition to comparing European and African men, the nurses constructed a distinction between "us" (the nurses and sometimes also me) and "them" (the women patients). They established that middle-class or professional femininity is different from the femininity of their mainly working-class or peasant women patients. And indeed the class differences were apparent. Sister Kiroro, who had been hand-picked by the researchers to run Bestlands, had a profitable coffee farm outside the city and a child in an American university; in the Kenyan context, she was from the tiny upper middle class.[15] Grace, the family-planning nurse, was almost as well situated. Wamuuchi and Mary lived in Best-lands and were not quite as well off. Wamuuchi was married and plan-ning to move to a better estate where she would have her own house built. Her husband's blue-collar job in the formal sector, however, had recently become more sporadic and less well-paying. Mary was a single mother living near the health care center in a one-room cement build-ing without consistent electricity or a private water supply. She was bet-ter off than many of Bestlands' residents but had little hope of moving out of the working-class area in the foreseeable future. The other nurses were in circumstances similar to those of Wamuuchi or Mary. Since middle- and working-class people in Nairobi were seeing their stan-dards of living decline with the recent increases in inflation and the reductions in state food and health subsidies, the gap between the eco-nomic situation of most of the nurses and those of their patients was narrowing during this period.

Whatever their actual class position in material terms, Bestlands' nurses perceived themselves to be quite different from their patients. After we saw the patient quoted earlier whose husband, according to Mary, was the one to blame for the patient's genital-ulcer disease, Mary said to me: "She has been faithful and now she thinks about AIDS—that's why she is crying. Imagine being faithful to somebody who is not even bothered about you!"[16] With this exclamation, Mary marked an "us" and "them" distinction. This woman was in a situation that Mary and, she assumed, I could only "imagine." Although the story Mary told about this woman was a familiar one, repeated to me over and over about most of the married women patients, Mary expressed amazement at the woman's predicament. This amazement spoke of difference; this was not a situation in which Mary, she implied, would find herself.

Similarly, a comment that Sister Kiroro made established for her audience of two other nurses and me that there was both literally and figuratively a considerable distance between herself and "them," the married women she talked to at the clinic. "Women do not question anything. She [a woman patient with an STD] left the *shambani* [rural home/farm] because she is sick and was not getting better there. They are not supposed to ask questions. They live oppression from their hus-band."[17] This woman did not even live in the city; for a city person, *shambani* means not just farm but also village, backwater, place of peas-ants. This rural woman was representative here of "them," the peasant women who "do not question." The distance was expressed clearly in the sister's use of the pronoun "they." Wamuuchi repeated this con-struction when she complained that all "you" (she, the nurses, and I) can do is "encourage them [husbands, wives] to talk. . . . [But] Kenyans do not talk about sex; it is taboo to talk." She did not count herself among the Kenyans who "do not talk about sex"; all day long it was her job to do precisely that.

Another way the nurses expressed their "difference" from patients was by explicitly casting doubt on the truth of their stories or by expressing their distrust of certain patients. On a number of occasions, Wamuuchi suggested I should not believe everything that I hear a patient say. As Wamuuchi reported in one instance:

> The boyfriend says he is not sick so he refused to come and she still has pain in passing. . . . She knows AIDS has no treatment but she does not take any precautions. She [tells me that she] left the boyfriend when he refused to come to hospital. *We don't know how true it is.* She was treated before. She was told to go to pay and she disappeared. . . . She knows about AIDS, she says she will leave him because he might give her AIDS. *We do not know how true it is.* [emphasis mine].[18]

The nurses asserted that because of their difference, cast more particularly as their superiority and relative modernity, they needed to "protect" Bestlands' women from their own ignorance and from men. According to Grace: "They need us to protect them. When a woman comes in for birth control, we know often her husband isn't allowing this. We have to take care of her and so we give her a birth control that he can't see [such as an injection or an intrauterine device], and we take care of her."[19] Grace went on to say that in contrast, the nurses knew how to take care of themselves and didn't put up with men who gave them trouble. Mary also made this clear to me on several occasions, hiding neither her pity nor her disgust for the patients who, as she put it, "do not even use family planning!" This sort of maternalistic attitude was absent at Casino but was very thoroughly integrated into the culture of Bestlands Health Centre, which is devoted mainly to maternal and child health care and family planning.[20]

The line between "us" and "them" was not always clear, however. Sometimes the nurses also identified with their patients as women vis-à-vis "African" men. Wamuuchi exclaimed to me, "African men! If you give a husband condoms, they can even divorce you."[21] Here, Wamuuchi put herself and me in her patient's position. In relationship to "African men," we (certainly heterosexual, ideally married) women are all disadvantaged and powerless. Wamuuchi seemed to erase the distance she and the other nurses carefully constructed in other contexts; at moments, the bond of heterosexual sisterhood closed the gap created by class. At another point, Sister Kiroro exclaimed in frustration that "we are made so submissive!" and went on to explain in a way that suggested she might have had an experience similar to her patient's: "If you are suspecting the husband [has an STD], and the first person you talk to is his father, you talk about all the evils he [the husband] has done. The father asks, 'Weren't you treated for this disease? So don't make a mountain out of a mole[hill]. Go back [to your husband].' And this is the father you thought you could talk to!"[22] Her use of "you" rather than "they" seems surprisingly inclusive.

The ambivalence reflects the contradictions and tensions in how nurses confronted AIDS and the fact that AIDS in Kenya has become a global issue. The nurses were not "European," but they were modern and were educated about biomedicine. They were women, but their education and class position protected them from total domination by men. The researchers' model of HIV transmission, of African heterosexuality, did not include a place for women like the nurses—or allow, in fact, for the effects of class differences among women at all.[23]

The nurses' recognition that women might fall into more categories of heterosexuality than "mother," "wife," or "whore"—the main groups of the high-frequency transmitter model—reflected another way in which nurses' constructions of women patients diverged from those of the researchers. At Casino, I noticed that a few staff members were happy to blame prostitutes for AIDS and even to assume that many of their patients were prostitutes regardless of what the patients said of themselves. Most of the staff, however, expressed a more complex view of the kinds of heterosexual relationships single women with STDs might be having. Women with a boyfriend (*rafiki*) were different from women with several boyfriends (*marafiki*). Both were different from prostitutes. Casino's nurses also suggested that it was not as easy as the researchers' model implied to identify who was a prostitute and who was not.

Such views were also common at Bestlands. Nurses tailored their advice (if not their views of men) according to whether a woman was a wife, a single woman with a boyfriend, or, although rarely, a prostitute. Like the nurses at Casino, Mary, Wamuuchi, and Sister Kiroro perceived important differences in a woman's ability to protect herself from heterosexually transmitted infections. As the quotes given above suggest, "wives" could really do nothing about either their husbands' philandering or their refusals to use condoms. The nurses did not believe they could even suggest that wives take condoms or—and here they differed from the staff at Casino—bring their infected and infecting husbands in for treatment. Even if a wife were pregnant, the dangers to her of talking to her husband about sex, treatment, or condoms posed, it seemed, a greater risk to her health than HIV/AIDS or STDs.

Most of the women who came for antenatal care or for family planning were supposed to be wives.[24] The nurses were not hostile to unmarried pregnant women or unmarried women who had an STD, but they were much less sympathetic to such women's complaints about men. According to the nurses at Bestlands, again like those at Casino, unmarried women, women with a *rafiki* or with *marafiki*, had a control over their bodies that wives did not. Wamuuchi and Mary both counseled young women to leave the boyfriends who would not use condoms. The women told her, Mary said, that "their friends refuse, they [the women] can't use them." But Mary would not accept this, telling them, "He's not your husband, there is no reason to take this; you should go to the boyfriend who is willing to use it [the condom]."[25] I never observed an interaction between a nurse and woman patient who either identified or was identified by others as a prostitute. Sister Kiroro did tell me a story about her interaction with a young unmarried woman who had *marafiki*. Sister Kiroro said she was angry at this "girl," called her a prostitute, and warned her that she would become sterile if she continued to have *marafiki*. Here again, nurses' constructions of women patients and of heterosexual agency seem at least occasionally ambivalent.

The nurses' constructions of heterosexual inequality and particularly of marriage greatly affected their ability (as they saw it) or willingness (as the research project's staff viewed it) to implement what was intended to be an important part of the project. The project was to combine treating and managing STDs among women with an attempt "to treat their male partners . . . thus ensuring that [women] are less likely to acquire STDs in the future" (CIDA 1990, 10). Nobody, not even the researchers, thought that getting husbands or *marafiki* to come in to the health care centers for STD treatment would be easy. Even at Casino, where many men were treated, few were willing to admit they had come because their wives or partners had asked them to. Nurses there often told me with frustration that these men make problems for bookkeeping and even diagnosis. The nurses reported that if the men were just to say that their partner had been treated for something, the nurses would know what to treat them for.

The first strategy was to have nurses tell any woman diagnosed with an STD to bring in her sexual partner. Nurses were to suggest that the woman tell her partner that if he also got treated this would prevent complications in pregnancy and protect current or future fetuses. Before I arrived, the researchers had abandoned that ineffective strategy. Next, they tried to have the nurses take the responsibility away from the women and put it on themselves. The nurses were to give women a note in Kiswahili stating that "the clinic"—rather than the sick woman herself—requested the man's appearance. The woman would simply be the messenger.

The nurses did not find either strategy useful. They asked very few of the many married women they treated for STDs to bring in their husbands. Why? I asked repeatedly.

> I didn't ask her [to bring her husband] because the way she talked she does not even use condoms. She doesn't even use a family-planning method. She thinks the man is the boss![26] . . . This is why we have such a problem with contact tracing.[27] The husband is on *safari* [a trip] to Tanzania; he comes back and slept with her one night and he is off again. He is not with her. So you see it is very sad. . . . You can't tell them to separate. You just encourage them to talk about AIDS, talk about it, to stick to home, to stick to his wife.[28]

Based on their understanding of "African" heterosexuality and gender relations, the nurses believed—logically (and, no doubt, with some experience)—that it was too great a risk for women to tell their husbands they had been to the clinic and were diagnosed with an STD. Husbands might well choose to claim that the woman had had sex outside the marriage. Alternatively, husbands might hear their wives' stories as accusations of infidelity (which, according to the nurses, they were). Either way, the wives were sure to suffer. The husbands were very unlikely to come to the clinic in any case.

Mary, Wamuuchi, Roseline, and Sister Kiroro did on occasion suggest that their patients ask their partners to get treated. Roseline indicated to me that she felt she had to: "You have to tell her the truth. I tell her—you have to tell her 'according to the results of the blood taken from you this morning or yesterday we found some sickness in it but you should not be very worried because you can be cured. We will treat you and your husband for the welfare of both of you and the infant.' So they definitely understand."[29]

According to the records that Mary and Wamuuchi kept in the STD room, they treated between 20 and 40 percent of their patients' partners each month. Most of the women whom I heard being advised to bring their male partners in, however, were unmarried women with a steady boyfriend. Nurses perceived these women, as I noted earlier, to be more in control of their situations than wives and likely to be less physically, emotionally, or economically devastated if their partner voted with his feet and disappeared. Based on what I am sure were accurate records, I believe that some married women were advised to bring in their part-ners. I was unable, however, to get the nurses to explain to me how they decided which wives to push and which to leave alone on the sub-ject. The overwhelming consensus was that most wives of African men would run too great a risk by cooperating with the researchers' plan. The nurses were for the most part tacitly unwilling to contribute to this risk.

The nurses' conviction that they were largely unable to implement the partner-treatment plan exposes the contradiction between the bio-medical high-frequency transmitter model and the health care develop-ment agenda. The model fixes a homogenized African man as a vector and his wife as a victim. The development agenda assumes that women (but not men), armed with biomedical information and backed by the supposed legitimacy of the project clinic, should, can, and will success-fully challenge this sexual and epidemiological inequality in their indi-vidual intimate relationships. Where these two sets of assumptions meet, the question emerges: How can women, especially wives, leap from being victims to being agents with sufficient control over their own bodies and over their experiences of heterosexual sex?

Bestlands' nurses decided that in most cases biomedicine was not the answer. They confronted a gap between what was expected of them by the researchers, who came armed with a model of married mothers as victims of prostitutes and in need of an "integrated" medical treatment and a counseling program that would empower them to intervene in men's behaviors, and the nurses' own constructions of working-class Kenyan women, men, and heterosexuality. The nurses asserted to me that while treating women for STDs was good in itself, the sexual and gender relations they perceived to be common in the community, and indeed in "Africa," implied that most women could do nothing to change men's sexual or health-seeking behaviors.

Six

Drugs for Whom?
"African AIDS" in the Second Decade

> The implicit ethical imperative to provide the "best
> proven preventive" methods to trial participants, how-
> ever, should include social and behavioral interventions
> to reduce HIV risk behavior such as needle exchange
> programs, for example. The absence of the best proven
> preventive methods in a community is often an indication
> that persons at high risk for HIV infection do not have
> the political power they need to obtain those services.
> (des Jarlais 1998, 1431)

> In developed countries, it will be ethically required
> that individuals in vaccine trials who are found to have
> acquired HIV infection will be offered antiretroviral
> therapy, which usually dramatically reduces virus levels.
> If vaccines cannot achieve protection against infection,
> however, treatment with antiretrovirals will compro-
> mise the ability of the trial to measure the efficacy of
> the vaccine in preventing disease. . . . Because of these
> complications, determination of the protective efficacy of
> HIV vaccine candidates may only be possible in trials in
> developing countries where the resources are not available
> to provide antiretroviral drugs. (Bloom 1998, 167)

These two observations were published in the wake of yet another
crisis-within-the-crisis that AIDS presented nearly twenty years after
its discovery. They refer to the apparently new terrain on which international battles over the production and distribution of knowledge about
HIV would be taking place during the new millennium: drugs, vaccines, and the people and institutions that produce them. Scientists
have framed the new battles in terms of medical ethics. They are challenging each other and health care development experts in international
organizations to decide if there can be ethical "universals" applied to
every research problem and location as if the world were one large laboratory or if material inequalities between countries in need of solutions
to HIV/AIDS justify using different strategies to test those solutions
in different parts of the world.

The two quotations above highlight the fact that these debates are

126

about political power, not simply between rich nations and poor but between those infected with HIV, their governments and scientists, and the rest of the world. Des Jarlais and colleagues address the widely accepted ethical rule that all trial participants, whether they receive the experimental drug or only a placebo, are given or allowed access to all other "best proven" prevention and treatment practices while enrolled in the trial. They make the crucial point that the degree to which trial participants have access to such practices, and therefore the degree to which any controlled experiment can be considered ethical, depends upon how much political power individual participants and people with HIV as a whole have in the countries where a trial is to take place. Their point can be extended to apply to nation-states operating in the global economy. To what extent can the governments of poor countries command the resources they need to get, make available, and sustain "best proven" treatment and prevention practices?

In an essay otherwise supportive of scientists' proposals to conduct controlled trials of HIV drugs and vaccines in sub-Saharan African countries, Bloom pushes the ethical envelope still farther. He suggests that it is precisely because "developing" countries cannot or will not provide already proven HIV treatments to their citizens that, from scientists' point of view, such citizens are the ideal subjects for vaccine research. In Kenya, for example, vaccine researchers are not required to provide subjects with any prevention or treatment options (except for condoms) other than the experimental vaccine; if HIV transmission is prevented in such a situation, researchers can be confident that the vaccine is effective. In short, people who have the least political power in the world offer the purest[1] data in experimental trials. According to Bloom, this apparent paradox renders the ethical questions surrounding vaccine trials ultimately unanswerable. These are the new politics of AIDS at the turn of the century: Will those who provide the data benefit from the way the data is used, particularly from fast-improving but extremely costly HIV drugs?

Scientists began to map out this new terrain in the early 1990s. In November 1994, just over one year after I returned to the United States from Nairobi, the *Journal of the American Medical Association* published a report that has had major repercussions for AIDS politics and policy in Africa and other parts of the world. U.S. researchers announced the results of two clinical trials of the drug azidothymidine (AZT). Infants whose mothers received a series of AZT treatments during pregnancy, labor, and delivery and who got AZT during their own first months of life were over 80 percent less likely to become HIV positive than infants born to women who just got a placebo (Connor et al. 1994). The results of Edward Connor's study were so statistically and medically significant that the trials were stopped early. Women enrolled in the trial who had not yet given birth and who were supposed to have gotten the placebo were immediately given AZT.[2]

Even as they offered some much-welcomed hope, however, the findings reignited old debates about mandatory HIV testing. Over two-thirds of U.S. women with HIV were then and still are poor and unlikely to be under a doctor's care in the absence of, before, or even during a pregnancy. Anonymous surveys of blood samples of newborns indicated that far more women were infected than had previously been suspected and, what is more significant, than had ever been given an HIV test (Abercrombie and Booth 1997). In other words, at the time scientists learned that AZT could prevent babies from getting the virus, very few of the women whose infants would benefit from such treatment knew that they had HIV, much less that they should be considering AZT treatment. Politicians and pediatricians in cities such as New York, Atlanta, Miami, and Los Angeles, where most of the HIV-positive babies were being born, began campaigning to pass laws forcing all pregnant women to get an HIV test at their first visit to the doctor so that if positive they could be given AZT as soon as possible.[3] Some HIV-positive women activists whose babies had died and many HIV-negative women just beginning to advocate for children with HIV supported these campaigns. Most AIDS activists who remembered all too well the stigma and violence faced by HIV-positive people during the 1980s, however, opposed plans to force anyone to get an HIV test or to take a toxic and expensive drug such as AZT (Booth 2000).

With the help of the Centers for Disease Control and Prevention (CDC) and the National Institutes of Health (NIH), U.S. health officials were eventually able to remove the issue from public view and therefore from political discussions. Several states quietly issued policies that encouraged physicians to make HIV testing and AZT treatment standard care for all pregnant women.[4] The federal government stated that if such policies failed to reduce rates of infection in babies by at least 50 percent, testing and possibly treatment would be made mandatory (Parham and Conviser 2002).

But debates over how to stop mother-to-child HIV transmission have refused to go away, despite important and complicated changes in the context of the debate and in the actors involved. While officials at the national level were successfully playing down the significance of the fact that women being targeted for testing and treatment policies are the most politically and economically vulnerable part of the U.S. population,[5] AZT was again becoming a political issue at the international level. In 1997, the WHO, the CDC, and the NIH both jointly and separately funded clinical trials to compare the effects of AZT on mother-to-child transmission of HIV with the effects of a placebo in Kenya, Côte d'Ivoire, Uganda, Tanzania, South Africa, Malawi, Ethiopia, Burkina Faso, and Zimbabwe in Africa as well as in Thailand and the Dominican Republic (Marshall 1998a, 1998b). The announcement of these trials launched a transnational debate over two intertwined ethical questions. Could research that can no longer be conducted ethically in a wealthy country that is able to provide AZT to all HIV-positive pregnant women be ethical in a poor country? Do researchers from wealthy countries have an ethical responsibility to make AZT available to all women in their studies (that is, to both experimental and control groups) if those women live in a country otherwise unable to provide the drug?

The story of Kenya's struggle with AIDS from 1984 to 1994 can be reread through this as-yet-unresolved debate. It is the story of "African AIDS" in a global context right up to the first years of the new millennium. The AZT debate demonstrates the persistence, under changed scientific and epidemiological conditions, of the contradictory construction of "African women" as agents, victims, and reformers of heterosexual HIV/AIDS that organized AIDS discourses in Kenya during the epidemic's first decade. The debate also suggests that crucial aspects of the politics of gender and science that we have explored in this book have not been at all unique to Kenya or to the relationships between Kenya, Europe, and North America. Kenya's story can also now be reinterpreted as a story about origins, not of HIV but of the colonization of AIDS in Africa by a specific gendered model of its spread and control. Kenya provided transnational scientists and policymakers the ideal ground on which to formulate the model of gender and heterosexuality that now serves as the foundation for current projects of control elsewhere in Africa and in South and East Asia.

After Edward Connor and his colleagues announced the results of the 1994 study that is now known as AIDS Clinical Trial Group 076, ACTG 076, or simply 076, scientists in the United States and at the WHO started asking whether this drug could significantly reduce perinatal HIV transmission in places with much higher rates of infection in women of reproductive age. Although for several years the WHO had been saying that preventing mother-to-child transmission should be a top priority in Central and East African countries, neither the much-better-endowed national health agencies of the United States nor the mostly U.S.-based multinational pharmaceutical companies specializing in HIV treatments had expressed scientific or financial interest in the problem. On the verge of losing its AIDS program to the UN Development Programme, the WHO jumped at the opportunity opened up by the excited international response to the 076 findings. Several U.S. universities as well as France's national medical research agency responded enthusiastically to the call for collaborative transnational research. Initially, all of the studies in Africa, Latin America, and East Asia were designed to include a sample of HIV-positive pregnant women "controls" who would, following standard scientific protocols, get only a sugar pill or placebo in place of the AZT given to the rest of the subjects (Marshall 1998a, 1998b; Lurie and Wolfe 1997a). In the African studies, an estimated total of almost 2,000 women would be research subjects whose infants got no protection from HIV (Angell 1997).

On the face of it, multisite clinical trials of AZT seemed entirely justified. In 1997, nearly 90 percent of the world's HIV-positive pregnant women lived in sub-Saharan Africa; most of the rest lived in Latin America or South and Southeast Asia. Of nearly 600,000 new HIV infections in children that occurred worldwide in 1998, almost all were due to mother-to-child transmission that occurred in these parts of the world (de Cock et al. 2000).[6] In 2002, UNAIDS and the WHO estimated that almost 3 million African children were living with HIV/AIDS (UNAIDS and WHO 2002).[7] In 1997, the percentage of pregnant women with HIV in the nine African study sites ranged from just under 7 percent to 33 percent and showed no signs of stabilizing (U.S. Bureau of the Census 2002). Figure 6.1 shows the prevalence rates among pregnant women in these countries.

The need for some way to prevent mother-to-child transmission was clear and urgent. Europe and North America had a drug that could possibly protect up to 75 percent of the babies who would otherwise be infected before, during, or after birth. One U.S. AIDS research team involved in the African trials summarized the situation created from these two realities:

> The P[erinatal] ACTG 076 regimen and the clinical impact of highly active antiretroviral therapy have resulted in 2 distinct epidemics. In industrialized countries, impressive reductions in HIV-related disease and death have occurred, so virtual elimination of new pediatric HIV infections is feasible. By contrast, developing countries face increasing levels of infection, disease, and death due to HIV. Perinatal HIV prevention offers a tenuous link to bridge this gap, to apply some of the recent biomedical advances in a rational manner in developing countries, and to regain some of the

Country	Geographic Area	Prevalence of HIV (%)
Burkina Faso	Capital city	6.7
Ethiopia	Capital city	13.0–18.2
Côte d'Ivoire	Capital city	9.1–15.02
Kenya	Capital city	11.0–20.0
Malawi	Capital city	25.0
South Africa	Nation	16.0
Tanzania	Capital city	13.0–14.0
Uganda	Capital city	15.0
Zimbabwe	Capital city	28.0–33.0

Source: U.S. Census Bureau 2002.

Figure 6.1 Prevalence of HIV Infection among Pregnant Women, Selected Countries in Africa, 1997

achievements in child survival that HIV and AIDS have erased. (de Cock et al. 2000, 1181)

This group and others argued that it was unacceptable not only to keep the results of our scientific progress to ourselves but also to miss the opportunity to protect (or salvage) the international investment already made in the health of Africa's children in the form of nutrition, vaccines, and prenatal care programs.

Such justifications were not articulated by the trials' sponsors until later, however, when the participating agencies and researchers were stunned by Drs. Peter Lurie and Sidney Wolfe's attack on the trials that appeared in the world's top medical journal just a few months after the first trials had begun. The decision by Marcia Angell, editor of the *Journal of the American Medical Association* (*JAMA*), not only to publish this attack but also to write an editorial expressing her agreement with it caused an uproar in the United States and internationally. Two well-respected AIDS researchers, Drs. David Ho and Catherine Wilfert, quickly resigned from *JAMA*'s editorial board. They protested Angell's refusal to retract her claim that the African AZT trials were a repeat of the infamously racist Tuskegee Syphilis Study that rewrote American and international medical-ethics policies (Jones 1992). Angell resigned from the editorship shortly thereafter. Representatives of the CDC, the NIH, the WHO, and UNAIDS as well as a number of the scientists directly or indirectly involved in the trials wrote blistering letters to British and American medical journals defending the trials. David Satcher, the U.S. Surgeon General at the time, supported the trials and found himself very nearly out of a job as a result. Other scientists opposed to the AZT trials and eventually some nonscientist AIDS activists wrote in support of the views published in *JAMA*. African scientists participated on both sides of the debate.

What generated all this frankly hostile discussion? The issue certainly was not whether babies in Uganda, Côte d'Ivoire, and Kenya should be protected from HIV infection. No one argued that perinatal HIV transmission was unimportant or that Tanzanians or South Africans should not get effective treatment. No one directly expressed concern about the danger of the toxic drug to the possibly extremely compromised immune systems of Zimbabwean or Ethiopian women or about AZT's rather severe side effects. The debate hung instead on the design of the trials. According to Lurie and Wolfe, the demand that all studies in Africa, Asia, and Latin America sponsored by the WHO, the CDC, and the NIH include a control group of HIV-positive pregnant women (and the babies they delivered) who would be given a placebo in place of AZT was unethical and violated both U.S. and international guidelines for conducting experiments on human subjects (Lurie and Wolfe 1997a).

Critics charged that the appropriate time for placebo studies of AZT had passed. AZT had already been tested, approved, and put into wide use in Europe and the United States to prevent perinatal transmission. They argued that since researchers knew that more babies of control subjects would become HIV infected because they were not getting AZT, it was entirely unethical to conduct a clinical trial in which some women would not get the drug at all (Lurie and Wolfe 1997a, 1997b; Angell 1997; Edi-Osagie and Edi-Osagie 1998). Such a trial would not be approved in the United States, where clinical trials cannot ethically ask subjects to get less or worse treatment than they could get outside the study. If such a trial is unacceptable in the sponsoring country, it is, the critics insisted, unethical in the host country. In *JAMA* and in a subsequent letter to Secretary of Health and Human Services Donna Shalala, Lurie and Wolfe (1997b) demanded that AZT be made available to all women and that the clinical trials be stopped.

Almost immediately the CDC, the WHO, UNAIDS, and the NIH responded by saying that there were likely to be biological and behavioral differences between the 076 population and pregnant women in developing countries that justified using placebo trials in the latter. New populations require (or at least justify) new—that is, placebo— experiments, they argued. The agencies and other proponents of the trials went on to explain that the experimental treatment was different, too. The researchers wanted to know if AZT in lower doses given later in pregnancy and for a shorter duration after birth would still prevent transmission. They argued on this basis that they were not really testing an already-approved treatment; the different dosage system was something entirely new. As such, a placebo comparison was not only ethical but necessary. Moreover, it would be unethical to test the standard, or original 076, regimen because none of the countries hosting these trials would be able to afford its US$800 price tag per mother-infant pair. The regimens to be tested would be much cheaper; the possibility of being able to provide all Ugandan women with AZT someday was more important than whether a small sample of women and babies in the research project got only a sugar pill. A third, closely related, argument was that AZT was only "known, approved, and available" in the United States and Western Europe. It was not available in the host countries. In effect, proponents argued, the women who get a placebo in the study are getting the "best available" treatment in Uganda, South Africa, or Kenya (CDC 1998; McIntosh 1998).

The critics returned the fire. Why not compare the shorter regimen of lower-dose AZT to the 076 regimen rather than to a placebo? Surely the fact that such a design would require larger samples of women (and therefore more money, drugs, and time) to ensure statistical significance was a small price to pay for preventing the illness and death of so many babies destined to get a placebo. According to Lurie and Wolfe (1997a) and a growing number of others, the trials' supporters were simply trying to make an end run around the ethical absolute that all subjects of medical research must get at least the best available treatment and that neither national borders nor international inequality could stop the 076 regiment from being the best available treatment, period.

Supporters held firm. Edward Mbidde, a Ugandan scientist on that country's AZT research team, argued that quite simply the 076 regimen is not feasible in Uganda because the government is poor and because very few Ugandan women come for prenatal care early enough to receive the full regimen (1998, 155).[8] He argued that what would really be unethical would be to provide the 076 regimen to research subjects in a country where no other woman would ever be able to get that treatment. He accused critics of the trials of being "irresponsible" and of endangering African lives. Another writer charged the critics with "ethical imperialism" because they applied absolute standards that disregard "the realities of economic conditions in the developing world" (Bloom 1998, 186). Still other scientists asserted that the critics' moral absolutism must be replaced by "morally relevant considerations of context that are necessary for the specification of universal principles" (Benatar and Singer 2000, 825).

By 1998, both sides were able to claim some sort of victory. Just a few months after it started, and during the most heated and public part of the debate, the placebo arm (or control group) of the Ethiopian study was called off. Of course, the participants in the debate could not agree about why things had changed. In their letter to Donna Shalala condemning the trials, Lurie and Wolfe implied that the Ethiopian study had been stopped because the Johns Hopkins University scientists there had realized that the research was unethical (1997b). Not surprisingly, however, spokespeople for the agencies funding the trials had a different explanation for the change in study design. The NIH's Lynn Mofenson explained that the Ethiopian study was redesigned by Johns Hopkins because an earlier placebo study in Thailand (the first of the trials to start) showed that the "short course regimen" of AZT was highly effective (McIntosh 1998). Joseph Saba of UNAIDS stated that without a placebo comparison, researchers in Thailand could not have gotten the results so quickly and been able to use the new regimen elsewhere (cited in Marshall 1998a, 1998b; see also UNAIDS 1999).

No qualitative or nonmedical studies of the operation or effects of any of these trials has been published. It is, in fact, fairly difficult to get clear information about what the trials looked like locally. This is particularly true in the case of Kenya, about which I have received conflicting reports, none of which appears in published form. Lurie and Wolfe list Kenya as one of the countries to host an AZT trial with a placebo arm (1997a). Peter Lurie told me in a personal communication that the Kenyan trial was funded by Belgium. This study was designed to test AZT and another drug, chlorhexidine, separately and in combination and to have one group of 250 women who would get a placebo (March 13, 2002). He too had been unable to find out whether the study was ever started and, if so, what its outcomes were. In a very brief news note in the *British Medical Journal,* Baraza (1998) states simply that the study designed for Kenya was never submitted to the national institutional review board for approval.[9] Searching for more, I contacted Kevin de Cock, a researcher in Nairobi who has written about perinatal HIV transmission issues. He reported knowing nothing about a trial of AZT either planned or carried out in Kenya.[10]

Whatever or whoever caused researchers to close down the placebo arms of their studies, the effect was to close down the debate over the ethics of research on perinatal HIV drug treatment. Today Kenya, like many African countries with high rates of maternal HIV infection, is struggling to get and distribute AZT and a more recently discovered drug known as nevirapine[11] to maternal and child health centers within their borders. AZT and nevirapine are repeatedly referred to by international health officials as "the only glimmer of hope" for Africa.[12] According to de Cock et al.:

> International agencies, donor countries, and pharmaceutical companies are helping establish pilot perinatal HIV-prevention projects in Africa, Asia, and the Americas, which will include thousands of women. The current core strategy is based on short-course zidovudine, with breast milk substitutes at birth or early weaning. (2000, 1177)

Although the research-ethics debate seems to have quieted down at the moment, the emergence, discussion, and apparent resolution of the AZT issue, like the "African origins" debates of the 1980s, continue to influence both international and local AIDS politics. The debate over conducting placebo research on AZT and nevirapine has been overshadowed by another set of debates. One argument is over the prices of newer, even more expensive, and much more effective drugs known as protease inhibitors. A second, closely related, debate is being waged over the responsibility and capacity of governments in poor countries to provide AZT, nevirapine, and other drugs for HIV treatment and prevention. The issues raised and decidedly not resolved by the placebo debate resonate in these currently contentious and explicitly globalized struggles.

At the 13th International AIDS Conference held in Durban in 2000, President Thabo Mbeki of South Africa shocked the world by stating that he did not believe that HIV caused AIDS. This statement derailed the conference. It also infuriated and mobilized activists, scientists, health care workers, and international AIDS and development bureaucrats. Although they have fought about many things, these groups shared complete confidence in the several decades of research demonstrating that HIV is the only consistent factor linking every known case of AIDS. The fallout from this statement has damaged Mbeki's international prestige and, more important, endangered the lives of South Africans living with HIV and AIDS. Although I in no way support President Mbeki's frankly irresponsible claim or his use of it to justify denying HIV-positive South Africans access to subsidized drugs, I believe that it is important to attempt to understand at least some of the reasons that he made this astonishing move.

In order to make some sense of what has been happening in South Africa and to grasp what its importance might be for efforts to cope with HIV and AIDS in sub-Saharan Africa, we should go back to several years before Mbeki's infamous speech. In 1997, the South African parliament passed a law allowing the state to import generic copies of patented drugs when the nation faced a health emergency. The parliament also defined the country's rapidly growing epidemic of HIV as such an emergency. For two years, the multinational pharmaceutical companies that own the patents on what researchers claim are the most effective HIV-related drugs put enormous pressure on the South African government to suspend this law. In 1999, the companies' efforts culminated in a lawsuit that claimed that South Africa was in defiance of World Trade Organization (WTO) rules protecting patent rights. Al Gore, then vice president of the United States, represented the pharmaceutical companies in a visit to Mbeki. Gore threatened to add trade sanctions to the lawsuit action in order to pressure Mbeki to change the law (Lewis 1999). Surprisingly, the South African state won the battle. Gore and the pharmaceutical companies were forced to drop the lawsuit and the threats when it became clear that the South African law did not violate WTO rules (Myers 1999) and when popular sentiment in the United States went against the drug industry.

The war was not over, however. In the same year, President Mbeki's health minister canceled efforts to launch a national program to administer AZT to HIV-positive pregnant women. She announced that the program was too expensive (Baleta 1999). Just a few months later, Mbeki announced that he had determined that AZT was highly toxic and too dangerous to administer widely. His statement at the AIDS conference doubting the "HIV theory" of AIDS came soon after (Baleta 2000, 1167).

The timing of Mbeki's announcement at the conference seems almost as strange as its content. By the start of the AIDS meetings, several of the multinational pharmaceutical companies—shamed by the international outcry against them and fearing further erosions of their patented profits—began cutting the prices of their most expensive drugs. Even with these cuts, most of the drugs remained far too expensive for the vast majority of people living with HIV in South Africa and other African countries (Swarns 2001). Still, the promises of further cuts prompted the governments of other African countries, including Kenya, to prepare their health care systems to distribute AZT or nevirapine to maternity hospitals and maternal and child health care clinics (Siringi 2001b, 133).

Mbeki's statement questioning the HIV theory backfired on him. Inadvertently the president strengthened the leading AIDS activist group in the country, the AIDS Treatment Action Campaign (TAC). Since 1998, the TAC's main objective has been to get free or very low-cost access to drugs that can prevent the transmission of HIV from mother to child, lower the amount of virus circulating in an HIV-positive person's body, and treat opportunistic infections resulting from HIV-related damage to the immune system. The TAC is now fighting on at least two fronts: against the multinational pharmaceuticals which continue to protest the loss of their patent profits (if not their rights) and against the president of South Africa.[13] Currently, one of the TAC's leaders, Zakie Achmat, is refusing all HIV treatment until drugs are made available to every South African who needs them. Nelson Mandela has emerged from his retirement to support Achmat and to criticize Mbeki, who was once Mandela's vice president.

How can we start to understand this situation? Why has Thabo Mbeki effectively abandoned the nearly one-third of his population now infected with HIV and the many more who will become infected? Without a great deal more research I cannot, of course, definitively answer this question. My analysis of the multinational biomedical project in Nairobi, however, leads me to wonder if Mbeki's challenge to the HIV theory of AIDS as well as to those promoting the widespread use of AZT to prevent HIV infection in infants might be read in multiple ways. It seems possible to reframe his rebellion as a challenge to the hegemony of a biomedical model that, while offering some hope of control and cure, has perpetuated racist and sexist representations and experimental "interventions" with dangerous consequences for many of sub-Saharan Africa's poorest people.

Thabo Mbeki has several times stated his belief that "poverty" is the main cause of AIDS, not HIV. While very problematic and indeed irresponsible on medical grounds, this statement makes sense if we read it as a comment on the global socioeconomic conditions that have nurtured the spread of the virus and determined the way that illness and death due to HIV infection is distributed around the world: over 90 percent of HIV-related deaths have taken place in the poorest regions of the world. Former U.S. vice president Gore and multinational pharmaceutical companies seemed committed to keeping it that way. To pretend that biomedicine, as internally complex and frequently helpful as it may be, has not been complicit in making this a reality is as dangerous and misguided as Thabo Mbeki's rejection of the HIV theory and of drugs that truly could help his people.

The new debates explicitly challenge the right of the international medical establishment, the U.S. government, and the U.S.-dominated WTO to define for Africans both the problem of HIV and the solution. These challenges are reminiscent of the earlier debate over "African AIDS." In the mid-1980s, many Africans voiced their anger at being blamed for causing and spreading the new disease. African leaders and journalists called Americans and Europeans racist and imperialist in a move to discredit claims that the disease originated in Africa, to challenge the right of foreign countries to expel African visitors, and to reject European and North American scientists' efforts to study the "African" version of the disease. Meanwhile, many African people were getting ill and dying (as they still are). The recent drug debates also confront the problems of racism in biomedical research and Africa's limited power over how transnational agencies and corporations construct African problems and "Africa" itself. The director of the USAID, for example, commented that he did not think "Africans" should get protease inhibitors because they were not capable of following the strict schedule for taking these drugs (Booker and Minter 2001).

The old and new debates are also quite different, however. In the mid-1980s, few Africans knew that they had HIV and fewer still were willing to start or join AIDS advocacy groups. Journalists, some local scientists, and politicians, not activists, politicized the problem. Now, nearly twenty years later, there are many groups advocating for rights, dignity, and care for people living with HIV and AIDS in every sub-Saharan African country hit by the epidemic. Many Africans have identified themselves as HIV positive in order to work for better care and treatment.

Moreover, unlike the early debates over "who started it," the debates over drugs and whether HIV causes AIDS emerge from the experiences and perceived needs of people with HIV or AIDS. Far from denying that there is a problem, participants in these debates address, albeit from opposing sides, the necessity of doing something concrete to stem the crisis. Although proponents of the AZT clinical trials declared that critics were just blocking effective interventions, all of the critics claim to want to get the already-proven treatments directly to every HIV-positive woman in Kenya and South Africa rather than waste time and, therefore, lives. Unlike the earlier struggles, the debates over drug research, patents, costs, and effectiveness assume the existence of the crisis and refer directly to the experience of actual people living with HIV/AIDS.

In many ways, the new struggles turn the debate about who gets to define AIDS on its head. In the very countries where African politicians had once told AIDS researchers to pack up their projects and go home, research participants are now demanding that those politicians and researchers give sick people access to treatment. Activists struggling for access to drugs do not reject Euro-American–dominated biomedicine. They claim instead that all Africans have a right to use its products. A condemnation of the practices of European and North American scientists remains, however. To the extent that biomedical scientists are complicit in the production and protection of drugs for profit, they are complicit in the deaths of Africans for whom antiretrovirals and protease inhibitors might have made a difference. By questioning the core assumption of biomedical knowledge about HIV/AIDS, President Mbeki has unwittingly made the contradictions and hypocrisies of the mainstream AIDS research and drug industry even more apparent.

So much remains to be understood and written about the history and politics of these most recent debates. By way of concluding this book, however, I want to focus particularly on what they can tell us about how the story of AIDS politics during the first decade of Kenya's crisis remains relevant to the analysis of what has happened since and to suggest what could happen in the future. Unfortunately, my reading of these debates suggests that the main lessons are about lost opportunities.

The international debate over whether the post-1994 placebo trials of AZT were necessary or ethical expose what is for me the most important of these lost opportunities. The decisions to launch these trials, the process by which the decisions were made, and the institutions that were involved in making them point to the persistence and power of a specific view of African women and, thus, the failure of officials, scientists, advocates, politicians, and feminists to seize the opportunity AIDS has offered to reorganize heterosexuality.

By itself, the enthusiasm of the WHO, UNAIDS, and their national counterparts in the United States about AZT as a means of preventing the transmission of HIV from infected African mother to African fetus or infant might be enough to make us wonder about these agencies' views of African women. The clinical trials proposed were designed exclusively for the purpose of assessing AZT's ability to protect fetuses and infants from their mother. Despite the fact that when taken alone or in combination with other drugs, AZT and other antiretrovirals can help people with HIV fight off opportunistic diseases attacking their own bodies, the 1997 initiative included no study of the effects, positive or negative, of AZT on pregnant or lactating women. The research designated pregnant HIV-positive Ugandan, Malawian, and Tanzanian women only as "vectors" of HIV to babies. Saving babies and protecting child-survival programs were the explicit and only goals. It has frequently been the case that even brief exposures to AZT for the purpose of protecting a fetus can make a woman biologically resistant to the drug, rendering it useless as a treatment for her own illness. Saving babies from a viral infection that is very likely to result in long, slow, and very painful deaths for them is unquestionably a good thing. But if one is saving them only to have them join millions of other orphans of women who are dead from the same infection, the validity of the project becomes less certain.[14]

The assumptions underpinning the experimental design of the research provide still clearer evidence that a specific construction of African women is at work. The WHO, UNAIDS, the NIH, and the CDC gave researchers a basic research design that required the use of a placebo group. Researchers and their institutions almost unanimously but entirely silently consented to this rule—put forward by the most powerful medical agencies in the world. This acceptance reinforced the "taken for granted" status of this particular research design. Layered with the fact that the research goal was to use women's bodies as a conduit through which treatment could be passed to fetuses, this design neatly fits with a certain view of African women. The persistence and widely shared character of an assumption that African women are simultaneously desperately in need of help and the cause of the worst possible aspect of the whole epidemic—dead babies—are at least in part what made it possible for agencies, researchers, and governments to take for granted that there would be no significant resistance to this initiative or to the fact that it remains so far the only systematic multicountry research on treatment for HIV infection.

One observer of the debates commented recently that the AZT trials positioned pregnant African women, and their governments, in a situation analogous to that of low-wage workers in *maquiladoras*, the sweatshop-like factories placed by export-obsessed governments and multinational corporations in poor regions of the world. Just as it may seem better to the government of a poor country to have bad jobs that damage workers' lungs and prevent workers (often violently) from unionizing than to have no jobs at all, it may seem better that "750 women" get AZT because of the trials than that no "poor women in Abidjan" get AZT at all (Schick 1997). Although the analogy is not perfect, the point is important. It highlights the problem of running clinical trials in a context where there is no alternative treatment, no promise and, as we know now, no likelihood of any future or long-term benefits to the women, their babies, or their communities from the trial. Nearly six years after the African trials were stopped, none of the countries hosting the trials is widely distributing AZT or nevirapine, let alone more women-friendly treatments.

Frequently there is no counseling or support for women who are identified as HIV positive by or during their quest for treatment for their babies. Dr. Dorothy Mbori-Ngacha is a Kenyan woman working with the multinational vaccine-research project based in Nairobi and a supporter of perinatal drug treatment. In an interview on the Web, she discusses how women's social situations and the failure to present treatment within a broader context that recognizes these situations affect the way women will interpret antiretroviral treatment:

> Over half the women accept testing, but less than a third of those who test positive come back for the interventions. We are trying to understand this. Why would you not return, after going through this whole process, to benefit from what we promised in the beginning? When women come to the antenatal clinic, their agenda isn't to learn their HIV status. They want antenatal care. They may get tested, but if it comes out positive, many aren't ready to deal with that. Many are afraid.
>
> I think we did it backwards, in a sense. We should have mobilized the communities so they would support a woman in using antiretrovirals for preventing transmission or for not breastfeeding her baby. Right now there isn't enough support. Her mother-in-law will ask and visitors will ask, and it will be very difficult for her to justify why she's not breastfeeding. (IAVI 2001)

Mbori-Ngacha avoids the question of whether researchers, governments, pharmaceutical companies, or international health agencies are responsible for this lack of community mobilization or support for women. Her frustration, however, suggests that it may be above all what is missing locally as well as globally—real support for women and particularly for HIV-positive women in sub-Saharan Africa—that makes AZT trials and their proponents' assumptions that African women should and will sacrifice everything else to save their babies and contribute to scientific progress truly unethical.

Like the research on prostitutes and mothers in Nairobi, neither the AZT research nor the subsequent (and at best half-hearted) efforts of the Kenyan, South African, and Ugandan governments to procure cheap versions of the drug have emerged out of discussions with affected or infected women themselves about their needs. Are limited health care funds best spent on AZT and breast-milk substitutes? Has anyone asked nonpregnant HIV-infected women what they need? How likely is it that governments and donors will support prevention efforts that address male sexuality and reproductive responsibility if their focus remains on stopping transmission in the womb or during birth? What other concerns, questions, and needs do HIV-positive women and women at risk have?

The current debates over drug prices and patent restrictions do not yet offer real hope that international or national health officials, scientists, or even activists will either listen to African women living with HIV or rethink their own assumptions about African women. Neither advocates for a radical restructuring of global trade relations nor, less surprisingly, defenders of the status quo are asking questions about who will get the cheaper (but never free) drugs and how. Given the fact that men's incomes are significantly higher than women's incomes all over Africa and that men are more likely to go to the private STD clinics where at least some drugs will be more available than they are in public clinics, it is reasonable to expect that men will get new treatments first. If there is any fear that new drugs might reduce the effectiveness of drugs used to prevent mother-to-child transmission, moreover, it would hardly be surprising if women's access to treatment for themselves were restricted.

The related debacle in South Africa over Mbeki's rejection of the HIV theory also points to lost opportunities. Conceivably, the mainstream AIDS research community could have from the start linked biomedical strategies with struggles to reduce African debt, end the World Bank and the IMF's inhumane economic restructuring activities, and mobilize especially poor and working-class African women against class, race, and gender oppression. Had it done so, I suspect we would be seeing quite a different political situation and a great deal less infection, illness, and death on the subcontinent.

These debates also expose the more hopeful or potentially positive side of globalization. They remind us of the possibility and effectiveness of localized but globally interconnected challenges to seemingly overwhelmingly powerful transnational actors. The debates also indicate that the postcolonial state in Africa, which is often presumed dead, is still important and not monolithically subservient to multinational corporations or U.S. interests. Many sub-Saharan African countries, including Kenya, have joined the effort to end patent restrictions and price controls over drugs. Together they have had some impact. The WHO, which initially was quietly supportive of the WTO, has now officially recognized and sanctioned the production, trade, and use of generic copies of a number of crucial HIV drugs.[15] U.S. pharmaceutical companies were forced by activists and eventually by public opinion to drop their lawsuit to stop South Africa from importing generic drugs. Kenya appears poised to win a similar battle (Siringi 2001a). Apparently when a state refuses to buy patented drugs, the capacity of transnational economic institutions to punish it is limited.

Even Mbeki's frightening stand on HIV has had positive side effects. It has strengthened and increased the grassroots base of the TAC. It has also created transnational solidarity around HIV-prevention and -treatment issues. U.S. and European activists have finally awakened; they have been forced to see the links between their struggles and those of their African sisters and brothers. These challenges and the varied responses of transnational actors to them suggest that globalization is not simply a top-down process. Using AIDS to mobilize broad support, some Africans have created at least a temporary coalition and have had what may turn out to be a lasting impact on the global economy. They have energized and are helping to capitalize the fledgling national pharmaceutical industry of another Third World country (India) and are discussing the creation of an African drug industry.

It is easy to exaggerate this success or to read it as a sign of African empowerment. The South African government has a legitimacy, wealth, and influence not possessed by Kenya, Malawi, or Côte d'Ivoire. It is very unlikely that on its own Kenya could have gotten away with disobeying the WTO and thumbing its nose at the multinational pharmaceutical industry. It is hard to imagine the Kenyan government attempting such a challenge, in fact, given the extent of its dependence on the United States and the World Bank. It is also true that South Africa's success was aided in no small way by the fact that activists and doctors around the world were already mobilizing support from human rights organizations in the United States and Europe for their argument that the WTO rules were unjustly killing Africans. On other equally important but less easily popularized life-and-death issues, such as charging fees for health care, countries such as Kenya have been unable to stop the transnational agencies from imposing policies that hurt the majority of citizens. Moreover, Mbeki's hard-line stance continues, together with severe economic crisis, to kill hundreds of South Africans every day.

The debates over these trials articulate the local, bodily experience of HIV infection and global processes in both familiar and new ways. The WHO and UNAIDS devised a single, essentially unvarying, model of research and intervention and applied it as a standard across many different countries and organizations of sexual and gender relations. When preliminary results of one of the studies came in, the new globalizing technology of the Internet connected researchers, funding agencies, and pharmaceutical companies, enabling a rapid reassessment of the original model. The Internet facilitated the rapid and wide distribution of new treatment recommendations. It also allowed me, by this time sitting at a desk far away from my fieldwork site, to follow the events and "read" the players and dynamics. At the same time, of course, groups such as Public Citizen, the TAC, and the AIDS Coalition to Unleash Power

(ACT UP) were using the same technology to find out what the agencies were doing, publicize their discovery, and mobilize support for their criticisms.

I cannot assess from here how most local-level health care workers in Nairobi are dealing today with the contradictions of this worsening crisis. Rates of infection have declined only slightly. Severe shortages of basic drugs and medical supplies persist, despite some improvements in the country's overall economic indicators. Thus far, activists, scientists, and officials involved in the debates over drug research and drug costs and access have passed up the opportunity to use this conversation about globalization, this repoliticization of the inequalities organizing the AIDS pandemic, to address sexual and gender inequality.

To assume that women in Africa are sexual beings with desires, goals, and strategies of negotiation is to challenge ideologies about masculinity, femininity, sexuality, and medicine that have been in formation since contact and colonization. It is to challenge the widely held and deeply entrenched assumption that women's sexuality is or should be exclusively about reproduction (of babies or of daily survival) and therefore always open to interventions from individual men, the state, and foreign experts. It is above all to challenge the notion that heterosexual men, across race, class, and national differences, do and should hold in common the control of heterosexuality, heterosexual desire, and rituals of heterosexual intercourse. In short, it seems there is little capital to be generated for the powerful by rethinking sexuality along these lines.

I imagine, however, that nurses at Casino, Bestlands, and clinics like them in Johannesburg, Kampala, Lilongwe, Abidjan, and Lusaka continue to struggle first and foremost with the problematic of gender, actively and alternately interpreting, reinforcing, and challenging the definitions of heterosexuality, femininity, and masculinity that they receive from ministers of health, researchers, donors, and patients. If research is to be useful and to contribute to a productive reframing of knowledge about HIV, one strategy might be to assist health care workers in evaluating the validity of, and then building upon, their own perceptions of women's opportunities to change heterosexuality.

Historically and ethnographically grounded critiques offer those of us who are frustrated by the limits and failures of "normal" science the opportunity to tweak its basic assumptions, to start to ask at least slightly different questions. Could the nurses' distinctions between wifely sexuality and the sexuality of single females guide epidemiological research or the selection of samples for microbiological study? Could we assume that women negotiate relationships that approximate as much as possible their own visions of what is satisfying, sexually and otherwise, without forgetting that they have significantly less power than men over the rituals and outcomes of heterosexual intercourse? Could the negotiations that unmarried women may engage in to get the sex they want (and avoid the sex they don't want) be as medically relevant as the choices that prostitutes make about asking clients to use condoms? Could the sexual experiences of single women be used in a positive way to talk to husbands about negotiations with their wives? Responses to these and similar questions are likely to be, as Nairobi's nurses have demonstrated, counterhegemonic, unpredictable, and challenging. Perhaps they can point us not only toward new strategies of HIV prevention but toward more long-term strategies for reinventing gender and sexuality in Kenya, Africa, and maybe even globally.

Notes

1. Global Medicine, Local Sex, and Crisis

1. "Bestlands" is a pseudonym. The names of the health care workers employed at the two clinics I studied are also pseudonyms.

2. The term "sister" comes from the English nursing system, in which all senior nurses were referred to by that term. Kenya has officially changed to the nomenclature used by the U.S. nursing system. In the clinics, however, nurses used the older terminology. The "sister-in-charge" is sometimes called the "matron."

3. I was able to understand the conversations that took place in Kiswahili as well as the ones that took place in English. I had to have translations of the conversations that were conducted in Kikuyu, the first language of Kenya's largest and most urbanized ethnic group and of most of the nurses at Bestlands. My inability to understand Kikuyu posed a problem for me in both clinics, where it was frequently used. Since I was also unable to use a tape-recorder in the field, I had to rely heavily on the busy nurses' typically (and understandably) quick summaries, which may not have accurately represented the patients' own words. The problem is mitigated somewhat by my not-coincidental decision to focus on the nurses' interpretations rather than on those of the patients. I cannot know how much of what the nurses actually said to patients (rather than what the nurses told me they said) I missed.

4. Author's fieldnotes, May 10, 1993.

5. Ibid.

6. "Special Treatment Clinic" and "Casino" are not pseudonyms. This clinic is both unusual and well known; it would be impossible to disguise it by

changing its name. The names of all of the health care workers here are pseudonyms, however.

7. Author's fieldnotes, February 26, 1993.

8. I put "African" in quotes here to indicate the problematic nature of the nurses' and the foreign researchers' use of this term to talk about Kenyans of any ethnic background living in Nairobi. This term was used by the colonial rulers as a catchall term for "black," "native," or "colonized peoples." When one is discussing sexual, economic, political, or other social practices of the vast majority of people who live on the subcontinent, it is depressingly common (in the United States particularly) but wildly misleading and, indeed, racist, to assume or assert any kind of continental (or racial) homogeneity. Thus, African scholars such as V. Y. Mudimbe (1988) have written about "Africa" as an invention by European and American scholars in the same way that Edward Said (1978) has written about the creation of "the Orient." Where I use the term "African" to describe any person or practice, I am alluding to this Euro-American construction. For the sake of easier reading, I have removed the quotation marks except where I want to emphasize the ideological aspect of the term; they are, however, always implied.

9. For discussions of these issues in African contexts see particularly Schoepf (1988 and 1997), Outwater (1996), Wallman (1996), Setel (1999), and Buvé, Bishikwabo-Nsarhaza, and Mutangadura (2002).

10. For examples see Baylies, Bujra, and the Women and AIDS Group (2000), Delacoste and Alexander (1987), and Schneider and Stoller (1999).

11. At Bestlands, which provided family-planning as well as STD- and HIV-related services, the nurses responsible for delivering family planning explained that many women want to use the injectable contraceptive Depo-Provera, the implanted contraceptive Norplant, or the surgically inserted intrauterine device (IUD) so that their husbands or partners would not know that they were using birth control. Nurses also helped their patients hide their contraceptive use by allowing them to leave at the clinic the appointment cards patients normally take home with them.

12. As in many other places where the United States used a fear of communism to justify supporting anti-democratic regimes, Kenya was never in any danger of becoming communist. Its first and second presidents embraced American-style capitalism and class inequality from the moment their country achieved independence from Britain in 1963.

13. Carole Joffe (1986), Darlene Clark Hine (1985), and Susan L. Smith (1995) have carefully documented the various and often-contradictory ways in which women nurses in the United States negotiate their own identities and beliefs about femininity in relation to women patients while simultaneously representing the state, private funding agencies, and biomedicine. Shula Marks's (1994) wonderful history of the nursing profession in South Africa takes up related questions but focuses on how black

and white nurses under apartheid struggled with each other and with the state over professionalization, class position, working conditions, and patient care. My thinking about the nurses as agents of the state is also influenced by Nancy Fraser's discussion of the "therapeutic" state (1989). In a largely theoretical essay on the "politics of needs" in welfare states, Fraser suggests that social workers, nurses, teachers, psychologists, and others actively (if not consciously) work to reorganize citizens' behaviors and identities—that is, citizens' perceptions of what they "need" from the state—in order to make them compliant subjects. At a very general level, finally, I am influenced by Michel Foucault's analysis of the clinic as an apparatus of the modern European state (1973 and 1977). Foucault argues that the rules and architecture of the public clinic serve the modern capitalist state by disciplining citizens' bodies, normalizing the "healthy" and defining the "diseased" as a distinct group to be controlled by the state via the clinic. Feminists have rightly criticized Foucault for ignoring the agency of actual people, such as nurses, and the possibility that they may not always follow the "rules." I think Fraser's discussion of nurses as representatives of the therapeutic state is similarly flawed. Nevertheless, both theorists insist that we can understand the state only as a set of disciplinary practices taking place in concrete local settings. This is a useful starting point for a study of nurses as political actors in national and global regimes.

14. The nostalgia for "home" has also, however, fueled many struggles organized by oppressed peoples to gain national independence, to enforce certain so-called traditional practices (often at a cost to women in particular), or to protect specific environments. Massey herself does not explicitly take this up; she focuses instead on the connection between this nostalgia and class, gender, and national privilege. But many feminist accounts of how women are configured in nationalist movements and are used by nationalist men provide evidence of this. See Afshar (1987), Yuval-Davis and Anthias (1989), Layoun (1991 and 2001), and Grewal (1996), to name just a few.

15. Since Annette Fuentes and Barbara Ehrenreich coined the term "the global factory" in 1983, feminist social scientists have been paying a great deal of attention to the relationship between gender and patterns of geographic dispersal of the process of producing a single good, such as a shirt, a car engine, or a computer (Fuentes and Ehrenreich 1983). Changes in production technology that have made such dispersal possible have allowed the most labor-intensive segments of the production process—which also usually happen to be the most dangerous segments—to be performed by the world's cheapest and least-organized workers, women of color. For an excellent recent review of this work, see Poster (2002).

16. Suspicions about the ability of ethnographic fieldwork to lead us to valid generalizations about social relations run especially deep in sociology. Mainstream sociologists have typically seen ethnography as at best capable of making survey instruments a bit more sensitive to "local" terminologies

and norms and as at worst a time-consuming and expensive obstacle to getting data on which mathematical operations can more legitimately be performed. The ethnography has long been the defining method of cultural anthropology, of course. As a result, anthropological discussions of its "validity" and "generalizability" have been much more nuanced and generous than they have been in sociology. Nevertheless, the method was invented to discover the boundaries of a given culture and was premised, therefore, on the assumption that such boundaries really exist, are relatively fixed, and fully contain the lives and experiences of the subjects under study. Certainly ethnographers have examined and challenged these assumptions over the years.

17. Moi and KANU claimed that "democracy" was not new to Kenya. Because citizens voted every so often, Kenya had been a democracy since independence; it just happened to be that sort of democracy in which citizens were allowed to "choose" only one party and, often, one candidate. Since 1992, Kenya has officially been a "multiparty" democracy. In reality, until 2002, it has been more accurate to refer to Kenya as a multiparty state rather than as a democratic state because although Kenyans voted and could, in theory, choose from among more than one party, their efforts to mobilize and to speak about serious opposition were still severely, often violently, repressed. The result of the 2002 elections, which seemed to have been run with little corruption, have given many Kenyans much greater hope. Moi stepped down with little violence (if you discount the civil war he fomented for more than ten years). His handpicked successor, also the son of Kenya's first president, Jomo Kenyatta, lost the election to Mwai Kibaki, the leader of the main opposition party. Kibaki's vision for Kenya, his views on AIDS, and his ability to negotiate with and within global capitalism are as yet not clear.

18. This report was neither published nor publicly distributed. Apparently this was because the USAID wanted to avoid angering the president, who was backing much lower estimates of HIV's prevalence. Although many people working on HIV in Nairobi had heard of the report, few had seen it. I was lucky enough to have a bootlegged copy slipped to me by a Kenyan friend with connections in the expatriate donor community.

19. Janet Bujra and Carolyn Baylies note: "Some AIDS campaigns in Africa are now beginning to target men, but they are often confined to condom promotion and personal risk awareness. . . . They appeal to men's self-interest rather than challenging their power over women or promoting mutuality between the sexes" (2001, 18).

2. Nairobi's Casino

1. Throughout the book I follow Kenyan usage and refer to all people in the country with white skin either as "European" or *Mzungu* (from Kiswahili; pl. *Wazungu*) unless I am referring to a specific person's or group's actual

nationality. The terms "European" and "*Mzungu*" refer to white people from the United States, Canada, and Australia as well as from Europe and Kenya itself. All the Kenyans who knew me knew that I was from the United States. Unless they were specifically asking me about "what America is like," they referred to me as a European or *Mzungu*. This usage is clearly a legacy of colonialism. In the sections of the book where I discuss colonial Kenya, I use the term "African" to refer to the indigenous peoples of Kenya because that was the official term, at least during the later years of British rule. In the rest of the book, except when quoting or paraphrasing a Kenyan who uses the term "African" to refer to a Kenyan with black skin, I refer to black Kenyans as Kenyans. I also use interchangeably the terms "Asian" and "Kenyan Asian" to refer to the members of the actually quite varied communities of people who themselves or whose families were recruited from South Asia by the British. They came initially to work on the Kenya-Uganda Railroad, to staff the lower levels of the colonial administration, and to open the small stores that European and Kenyan consumers alike would come to depend on. Throughout East Africa, the Asian communities became both a class and racial "buffer" between European and African. For a discussion of these communities, see Gregory (1993).

2. Obudho and Aduwo add that women were underrepresented in the European community in Nairobi. In 1962, the sex ratio among Europeans was 116 men to 100 women (1992, 60). There is every reason to believe that it was even more skewed before independence; *Wazungu* women were not encouraged to come to the city until the government recognized the need for European nurses and social workers after World War II (Lewis 2000, 284).

3. For the origins of this argument, see Wolpe (1972) and Meillasoux (1975, cited in Cooper 1983, 9).

4. White (1990) found that a significant number of the mostly Kikuyu women who migrated to Pumwani soon after it was established built or bought houses which they then rented, again usually along with other, more intimate, services, to male workers. Most municipal officials turned a blind eye to these prostitutes until the end of World War II. This form of settled prostitution, White argues, was tolerated in fact (although reviled in rhetoric) because the city government was not willing to spend its own money on housing or services for Africans.

5. For an important discussion of the blaming of prostitutes for syphilis in imperial London, see Walkowitz (1980).

6. A full discussion of colonial racial and sexual ideology is beyond the scope of this chapter. Fortunately there are a number of excellent accounts of the development and content of "racial science" as it circulated between Europe and its colonies. See, for example, Stoler (1991), Schiebinger (1993), Fausto-Sterling (1995), and various essays in Harding (1993) for important feminist accounts. For discussions of the contradictions and conflicts in the racist thinking of whites in Kenya in particular, see Kennedy

(1987), Shaw (1995), and Maughan-Brown (1985). On the closely related constructions produced by settlers in South Africa, see Comaroff (1993). On European and North American constructions of "Africa" in popular culture, see Nederveen Pieterse (1992), Lutz and Collins (1993), McClintock (1995), Watney (1989b), and Gilman (1985 and 1988).

7. For discussions about the relationship between imitation and the European production of the identity of the colonized, see Homi Bhabha (1984) and Tania Modleski's feminist reinterpretation of Bhabha (1992). Drawing on the work of Frantz Fanon, Homi Bhabha has argued that colonial discourse produces—or expresses the colonizer's desire to produce—a colonized subject who wants to be and becomes like (dresses like, speaks the language of, reads the books of) the colonizer but who can never actually be the colonizer. The fully colonized subject unconsciously becomes, in the eyes of the colonizer, a mimic; that is, a good but incomplete and often-laughable imitation of the colonizer. In the postcolonial world, the colonized mime ultimately becomes an inferior replacement for the colonizer; he functions to undermine efforts by the colonized to achieve true political and psychic independence. Modleski reworks this argument by suggesting that while racist ideology requires the colonized to imitate (inevitably unsuccessfully) the colonizer, sexist ideology transforms women into (always-failed) imitations of men's desire. Both Euro-American women and African/African-American men own some piece of the colonizer's claim to power. Women of color, however, share nothing of the Euro-American man's embodied superiority. They will never be able to erase the distance between their real selves and those whom they are expected to imitate. Representations of African and African-American women's sexuality in American popular media, she concludes, most completely and, for the colonizer, most satisfactorily, reflect the colonizer's desire for embodied, simultaneous, and inextricable sexual and racial domination.

8. Of course "the white man" would also have proven definitively that the African was inferior. As Ann Stoler (1989b), Londa Schiebinger (1993), and others have pointed out, imperial ideologies are fundamentally contradictory. Europeans did not always agree with each other. As early as the 1920s, the notion that Africans were little removed, biologically and morally, from apes had met with intense criticism from various quarters, including anti-imperialist activists in England, certain missionaries, sections of the British public who were grateful to Africans for their contribution to winning World War I, and the emerging leaders of nascent nationalist movements in Kenya and elsewhere in the empire. Conservative settlers, who were particularly interested in seeing that the colonization which had given them such wonderful farms and cheap labor was a permanent condition, continued to insist that Africans could never be as intelligent as any European child, much less capable of governing themselves. The paternalist perspective became gradually more accepted by members of his majesty's colonial civil service, particularly those astute enough to realize that

the British empire was unlikely to last for many more years. See Maughan-Brown (1985) for an interesting discussion of the contradictions of ideology among Kenya's settlers. See also Shaw's (1995) reading of settler accounts of Africans' "beastly" sexuality. Shaw suggests that even among settlers' representations, one can see these different views competing for primacy. Moreover, according to Shaw, settlers drew sharp distinctions between different ethnic groups within Kenya. In particular, the pastoralist Maasai were viewed as "savage" but noble. The Kikuyu, who formed the bulk of the labor force in settler homes and fields, were more likely to be seen either as childlike or as "ignoble" beasts.

9. It was always a he; the possibility of an African woman holding formal political power was never entertained.

10. Lewis (2000) notes that the fears of whites in the colonies paralleled ruling-class folks' fears in Britain that the poor, once mobilized against the enemy outside, might then turn against the enemy within. The postwar victory of the Labour Party seemed to justify these fears. Growing an extensive welfare state, however, required a compromise between left and right, socialist and capitalist, that ultimately proved to buttress capitalist development in the metropole. There are, of course, many accounts of this process in Britain and elsewhere in Europe as well as in North America. Lewis is the only one to have investigated the related, although of course hardly as extensive or progressive, process in East Africa.

11. See Dawson (1983) for a discussion of the colonial view that urbanization itself was "corrupting" the otherwise innocent African who should have been left alone in his bucolic, albeit backward, village. Also, see Shaw (1995) for a summary of white settlers' views that Africans who left the plantations for the city became irredeemably corrupt.

12. I have been unable to find a reliable document stating precisely the date that Casino opened. I am basing my estimate on those made by various people whom I interviewed in Kenya.

13. The British typically considered tribal or ethnic identity to be a crucial variable in their medical research on Africans. This reflected the official colonial political system of "indirect rule" in which "tribes" were supposed to organize local affairs. It also reflected the unofficial colonial system of divide and conquer. British assertions about "tribal" differences of biology and culture were often invented differences that were predicated, however consciously or unconsciously, on a determination to intensify and then use inter-African conflict to benefit the colonial regime and economy. Thus, a survey of syphilis among African women done in 1939 reported significant differences in prevalence by ethnic group. Forty-five percent of those with syphilis were "Swahili, Somali, Abyssinians and Sudanese" and Ugandans. Twenty-five percent were Nandi and Luo. Twenty percent were Maasai and Kamba. Ten percent were Kikuyu (de Mello 1947, quoted in Dawson 1983, 245). Why those reporting the findings grouped tribes the way they did is unclear, although singling out the Kikuyu, with whom the

colonizers had the most intimate relationships and who were most likely to live in or migrate to the city, was a common practice. The Kamba and Maasai, both of whom lived relatively near the city and near the Kikuyu reserves, were also fairly well known to the colonizers. Perhaps the first category was of people considered "foreign" to Nairobi.

14. See especially Allen Brandt's discussion (1987). Penicillin-resistant strains of syphilis and other diseases have forced biomedical and development experts to create new kinds of treatment regimens (Verhagen et al. 1971; Ronald, Plummer, and Ngugi 1991).

15. It is important to note that Lyall's report, while the only such text explicitly about Casino, does not reflect an idiosyncratic view of sexually transmitted diseases and the necessity of targeting African women to stop their spread. Similar views and proposals were presented by policymakers and researchers focusing on other cities. See particularly Meghan Vaughan's discussion of Uganda (1991, 130).

16. In the port city of Mombasa there is still an STD clinic in the hospital. Prostitutes are required by law to register there monthly. When they are pronounced free of STDs (not including HIV), they are given a green card that for the next month allows them to work. If a sex worker does not have a current green card, she can be arrested by a police officer or a city sanitation official and forced to attend the clinic. This clinic was created between World War I and World War II to protect foreign naval troops from infections. A history of this clinic remains to be written.

17. Author's fieldnotes, February 25, 1993.

18. Randall Packard (1989) was one of the very few scholars to publish the view that the sudden and rapid increases in HIV infection in Kenya and elsewhere in Africa might be explained not by "promiscuity" but by dirty needles, specula, and other medical instruments. Such views were, and still are, considered heretical by the biomedical community in the United States. See also Packard and Epstein (1992).

19. Discussion paraphrased in author's fieldnotes, March 2, 1993.

20. Not only do the groups overlap in membership, but people with ulcers and other symptoms of untreated sexually transmitted diseases such as syphilis and chancroid are also physiologically more vulnerable to being infected during intercourse with an infected partner. They are more likely to transmit the infection during sexual intercourse with others as well (Plummer et al. 1991).

21. Author's fieldnotes, February 25, 1993.

22. "Clinical officer" is the British term commonly used in Kenya to refer to the medical practitioner working in a clinic or health center who is trained to diagnose illnesses and prescribe drugs. The clinical officer may be a fully qualified medical doctor (MD) or an MD who has not yet completed his or her residency. Most commonly, however, the clinical officer has qualified for the position with significantly less training than an MD. She

or he is analogous to the American physician's assistant (PA) or nurse-practitioner (NP). In the United States, the PA and NP positions emerged long after the establishment of a cadre of medical doctors. In contrast, under British colonial rule, the clinical officer was the highest medical position that a colonized individual in Africa, Asia, and the Caribbean could obtain. This cadre was created by the British to staff "native" clinics for three reasons: first, so that European doctors would not have to have direct physical contact with the colonized; second, to avoid establishing expensive medical schools in the colonies or sending "natives" to Britain for medical education; and third, to delay the development of a "native" professional class whose members might perceive themselves to be the equals of their colonial rulers (Beck 1981; Marks 1994).

23. Author's fieldnotes, March 13, 1993.

24. Author's fieldnotes, March 4, 1993.

25. Chancroid is an infection that results in an acute ulcer ("soft chancre") on the genitals, often mistaken for syphilis ("hard chancre"), herpes, or other genital ulcers. It is caused by the bacteria *Haemophilus ducreyi*. Chancroid "is a sexually transmitted disease more prevalent in individuals from lower socioeconomic groups who frequent prostitutes" and in men who are uncircumcised (Ronald and Albritton 1992, 269). The Winnipeg outbreak is discussed in Hammond et al. (1980).

26. Author's fieldnotes, March 1, 1993.

27. The shortage of HIV-testing kits meant that the doctors, clinical officers, and nurses often determined that a patient had HIV if she or he had one or more symptoms of AIDS. Those patients who had skin lacerations, thrush, an STD that was not responding to treatment, or herpes zoster, a specific type of genital sore associated with HIV infection, were rarely given HIV tests because it was decided that the symptoms were indication enough of infection.

28. Author's fieldnotes, February 26, 1993.

29. Author's fieldnotes, March 17, 1993.

30. Author's fieldnotes, April 20, 1993.

31. The question of whether my function at Casino, or, perhaps, my payment for being allowed to do my own research there, was to "report" to the researchers or to the donors came up repeatedly. Initially I responded by saying that such reporting was not my purpose and that as a sociologist I was really not qualified to evaluate the procedures or personnel at the clinic. I was determined not to become a "spy" on the staff; several nurses asked me directly if I was there to evaluate them and I wanted to be able honestly to say "absolutely not." As it became clearer to me that both the matron and the research group were counting on me to give them something concrete before I left, however, I ultimately agreed to write for them a short summary of what I thought were some of the main issues or problems raised by efforts to counsel women patients about HIV/AIDS. I wrote my

summary several weeks after ending my fieldwork at Casino. I gave a copy to the matron and used it as the basis of a presentation to a class of public health students at the University of Nairobi. I never did give a copy to the research group or to the donors (although they certainly could have gotten it from the matron) because I wanted it to be clear that I was not working for them. Despite my efforts, I am quite sure that the matron never stopped associating me with the *Wazungu* doing research and planning renovations. She often asked for my advice on what I thought donors would be most interested in and on whether I thought her ideas were "good" ones. This is hardly surprising; the researchers had had several young white women graduate students join them to do the nonmedical studies that they were not interested in doing themselves. One Canadian master's student had developed a training manual to educate nurses about STD and HIV counseling. The two full-time health education and counseling people on the team were both white women just slightly older than myself. My race (and the assumed wealth that came with it), gender (and the assumed interests and roles that came with it), and education put me in the same category as these other women. This was somewhat difficult to negotiate, particularly since the research team had, and was perceived by the matron to have, enormous influence over the donors. From the matron's point of view, if I was connected to the team, then by definition I too had such influence. I am sure that at least during the first several weeks of my visit, the matron and the nurses who followed her orders were on their best behavior and were consciously trying to give me the answers they believed that I or the matron wanted. Probably the matron maintained this perception of me. I do not think that the rest of the nurses did to the same extent, particularly since it fairly quickly became obvious to them that I knew absolutely nothing about diagnosing or treating STDs (or anything else medical). My ability to speak Kiswahili well and the fact that I did not ride in the "research van" with the team but arrived at Casino alone and on foot also distinguished me from the research team and the donors. Nevertheless, of course, I was always white and therefore, I have no doubt, potentially powerful.

32. And despite the much-belated official acknowledgment in 1992 by the Ministry of Health that there were men who have sex with men, at least in the prisons and army.

33. It is important to note that it is very possible, in fact likely, that at least some of the staff did judge patients by their tribal affiliation. In Nairobi, countless sexual stereotypes attached to different tribes and communities circulate widely and are used to express feelings of superiority, to poke fun at, or to dismiss the people of other tribes. The official line in Kenya, however, is that there is no "tribalism" at all. As state workers, the clinic's staff members were unlikely to share their views of tribal difference with me or with other *Wazungu*. For a recent discussion of tribalism and tribal politics in Kenya, see Orvis (2001).

34. Of course, the context in which and the purposes for which "gender" is defined at any given moment are absolutely crucial.

35. Author's fieldnotes, March 3, 1993.

36. As a sign of respect, clinical officers were often, but not always, referred to as "Doctor," even though they did not have an M.D.

37. Author's fieldnotes, March 3, 1993.

38. Author's fieldnotes, April 1, 1993.

39. Ibid.

40. Author's fieldnotes, March 27, 1993.

41. Author's fieldnotes, April 3, 1993.

42. Author's fieldnotes, March 17, 1993.

43. Author's fieldnotes, March 13, 1997.

44. Author's fieldnotes, February 26, 1993.

45. "*Magonjwa ya zinaa*" literally means "diseases of fornication." Johnson (1984, 543) uses the terms "*mambo ya uasherati*" or "*uzinzi*" to translate "venereal disease" and has no term for "sexually transmitted diseases." "*Mambo ya uasherati*" translates literally as "problems related to or resulting from adultery or fornication."

46. Author's fieldnotes, March 13, 1993.

47. Author's fieldnotes, March 3, 1993. The Kikuyu are the largest ethnic group in Kenya. The overwhelming majority of Kenyans living in Nairobi are Kikuyu. Most of Casino's nurses are also Kikuyu. I had to have the assistance of translators to understand conversations between the Kikuyu nurses and Kikuyu patients. Discussions with patients from other ethnic groups or involving nurses from other ethnic groups usually took place in Kiswahili, which I could translate myself, or in English. The multiplicity of languages in Kenya and the fact that many Kenyans prefer not to speak Kiswahili makes doing ethnographic research in multiethnic Nairobi very difficult. I cannot know how precisely nurses or other translators actually translated the Kikuyu conversations for me; I suspect that much of the nuance was lost. Nevertheless, because I focus primarily on the nurses' stories, not the stories of the patients, I believe that whatever the nurses told me reasonably reflected their view of their position and their patients' position relative to me and to the researchers and other expatriates involved in the work at Casino.

48. Author's fieldnotes, March 3, 1993.

49. Author's fieldnotes, April 5, 1993.

50. Author's fieldnotes, February 26, 1993.

3. Negotiating AIDS Policy in Kenya

1. See Lutz and Collins (1993) for a different route to the same conclusion about images of "Africa" in American pseudoscientific media. For other

discussions of European and U.S. representations of African sexuality, see Schiebinger (1993), Nederveen Pieterse (1992), and Gilman (1985).

2. To be fair, under this headline is another that reads: "Coming to Terms: Residents of a Triangle HIV/AIDS Family Care Home Make Peace with the Past." AIDS is neither gay nor African, perhaps. It is also important to note that Van der Horst's article itself is not especially sensationalistic or "colonial." I focus here on the attention-grabbing headline that subsumes all of Africa (where HIV is very unevenly spread) under the term "AIDS-plagued." I do not know who chose the title.

3. Although they admit that Uganda's government has been a bit "better," apparently Uganda's president has not gone far enough to undermine the generalization.

4. One of the many problems of this formulation is the lack of geographical specificity. Does the "West" include Latin America, for example?

5. Lesbians of whatever nationality were not considered at all (Hollibaugh 2000).

6. At its first meeting, the WHO distinguished AIDS in Africa from AIDS in Europe and North America, suggesting there were two distinct "epidemiological patterns" of the disease: "In most western European countries and Canada, the epidemiological pattern is very similar to that in the United States, the majority of cases being in homosexual men. In other areas, such as equatorial Africa and the Caribbean, the pattern seems to be different, with no identifiable risk factor for the majority of cases" (WHO 1984, 419).

The characterization of the pandemic as composed of two distinct and static patterns—homosexual in North America, Western Europe, Australia, and New Zealand and, at first, mysterious in Africa and Haiti (see Farmer 1992)—was soon transformed into a global schema. In November of 1986, Jonathan Mann, two American scientists, and one Belgian scientist wrote an article on AIDS in Africa published in the widely read and semi-popular American journal *Science* (Quinn et al. 1986). This article elaborated on and further fixed the notion that there is a fundamental difference between African and North American or Western European AIDS. The article's title indicates the premise of Africa's "difference": "AIDS in Africa: An Epidemiological Paradigm." "African" AIDS was so different as to constitute a paradigm in itself. According to the authors, the way in which the virus works within the body is essentially the same for all people with AIDS, but the way in which it is spread from one individual to another and in which it eventually manifests itself as AIDS clearly and sharply differs between Africa and the United States. The initial marker of this difference was, according to these authors, the fact that among Central Africans living in Europe who were diagnosed in the early 1980s with AIDS, the ratio of men to women was 1.7 to 1 compared with a ratio of 16 to 1 among (white) "Europeans" and North Americans. Second, only 5 percent of the Africans said they were homosexual or bisexual, compared with 85 percent in North America. The African pattern is composed of the following characteristics: a roughly equal sex ratio, a young age (a mean of about 37 years old for men and 30 years old for women), bi-directional (i.e., female-to-male as well as male-to-female) heterosexual transmission occurring among those with a large number of sexual partners, single status and prostitution for women, and married status for men. It is the heterosexual promiscuity in Africa that constitutes the paradigmatic factor. For related critiques of the "pattern" model, see Farmer (1992, 142–143), and Setel (1999).

7. The Africans' communiqué went on to critique the hypothesis that the virus originated in African green monkeys and to question some European and North American researchers' assumption that the presence in Central Africa of Kaposi's sarcoma, a cancer identified in the United States as an AIDS-related opportunistic disease but long endemic to areas of Central Africa, indicated an African origin for the syndrome. The African representatives did not deny the probability of AIDS becoming a serious problem in their countries. In their statement, they requested "help to install safe blood-banks to minimalise the risk of AIDS being transmitted through blood transfusions. They also called for help in setting up cheap laboratory methods to diagnose the disease" (Chirimuuta and Chirimuuta 1989, 122–123). Given the racism they had confronted, it was remarkable how reasoned the Africans' response at the Brussels meeting was. In his summary of the media responses to AIDS during this period, however, Renée Sabatier (1988) notes that many African researchers, politicians, and journalists did react to racist blaming of Africa and Africans for HIV with often-homophobic counteraccusations against European countries and the United States.

8. In her most recent book, Cindy Patton (2002) points out that the WHO's early labeling of Asia as "low risk" is at least partly to blame for the fact that so little was done in this region until HIV had already become widespread. She suggests that the "pattern three" designation was premised on imperialist views of Asia and Asians as sexually passive. Unlike sexually aggressive (masculine) Africans who "naturally" started the whole problem, passive, docile (effeminate) Asians would remain unaffected or, at worst, join the pandemic very late. Recent reports of an HIV crisis in India make clear how misguided and dangerous this thinking was.

9. In 1987, the World Health Assembly asserted that the WHO would take "international leadership" in the effort to control the pandemic by adopting a two-pronged "national" and "global" approach. The Global AIDS Strategy presented the WHO as that body ideally situated in the international scene to manage the transfer of money and expertise to Africa by virtue of its status as a global technical agency (WHO 1987).

10. This last move reflected the WHO's Executive Board's concern that some member countries might not support the use of their contributions for control of the controversial disease and its expectations that developing a

successful AIDS program would be costly, that rich countries would be motivated to donate over and above their regular dues, and that efforts to mobilize AIDS funds could serve as a tool for educating policymakers about the crisis.

11. For a good, albeit uncritical, account of the WHO's massive and interventionist "vertical" smallpox campaign to which Mann compared his vision of a battle against AIDS, see Brilliant (1985).

12. Interview with author, April 17, 1992.

13. Author's interview with Priscilla Alexander, April 20, 1992.

14. The problem of maternal HIV infection, which was rapidly increasing among low-income communities of color in the United States, was nonetheless asserted to be a threat exclusively to Africa where (again conflating into a single statistic an extremely varied epidemic) "it is projected that by the end of 1992 about a million children will have been born to infected women; about a quarter of them will be HIV-infected, and most of them will die of AIDS" (WHO 1990c, 1).

15. Child-survival programs were very popular objects of donor money and even more of donor rhetoric for several reasons. One, they could be defined as "nonpolitical" while simultaneously opening up the state to rather intensive donor interventions. Two, they were a critical vehicle for population-control messages and measures; spacing and limiting births by using modern contraception was presented as key to improving the health of children. Third, they were a major strategy for "integrating" women into development. By offering child health care along with training in crafts, farming, and so on, development agents could draw women into these programs. Fourth, they were a relatively cheap way of improving the long-term health of Africans and hence reducing the economic burdens of adult illnesses on the economies. Certainly they went a long way toward popularizing biomedicine; immunizations really worked. And finally, they were an effective legitimating tool for donors; who could argue that international interventions for the sake of the child were "neo-imperialist evils"?

16. Interview with author, March 12, 1992.

17. As early as 1965, it was revealed in a euphemistic policy statement that while British and resident Indian staff (categorized as expatriate) were being expelled, expensive foreign experts were being brought in to supplement the rapidly deteriorating Africanized services (Himbara 1994, 117).

18. This is a rather simplified summary. There has been a great deal of interesting discussion and debate about both Kenya's "miracle" and its subsequent bust. In addition to the sources cited in the text, see Gertzel (1970), Leys (1975 and 1994), Langdon (1977), Kitching (1980 and 1985), Sandbrook (1985), Schatzburg (1987), Ford and Holmquist (1988), Barkan and Chege (1989), Bates (1989), Thomas-Slayter (1991), Berman and Lonsdale (1992), Holmquist, Weaver, and Ford (1994), Holmquist and Ford (1994), Ogot and Ochieng (1995), and Ahluwalia (1996).

19. The WHO consistently uses the word "invited" to explain its staff members' country visits. It is unlikely, however, that Kenya's minister of health, Peter Nyakiamo, simply and entirely voluntarily chose to invite Mann. Nyakiamo was certainly aware of his president's attitude toward AIDS, on the one hand, and, on the other, of the mounting pressures from scientists in Kenya, the tourism industry, and at least some foreign donors to join Uganda in allowing the WHO to set up a national program.

20. Interview with author, May 17, 1992.

21. Interview with author, May 25, 1992.

22. Most of the nearly US$3.5 million pledged to Kenya's National AIDS Control Programme (NACP) in July 1987 was pledged to Kenya by donor countries through the WHO/GPA's trust fund program. Eighty-two percent (US$2,855,750) was to come through the GPA from Denmark, Norway, the United States, the UNDP, and from the GPA budget itself. The rest, $640,000 (18 percent), was pledged directly to the Kenyan government by Belgium, the European Economic Community (EEC), and the Ford Foundation. The GPA contribution constituted 12 percent of the total donor contribution for 1988 and was the fourth largest donation after Norway (22 percent), the United Kingdom (16 percent), and the United States (14 percent), all of whom contributed through the GPA (Government of Kenya and WHO 1987).

23. Interview with author, July 12, 1992.

24. Interview with author, December 5, 1992.

25. Interview with author, July 12, 1992.

26. Interview with author, November 7, 1992.

27. Interview with author, July 12, 1992.

28. For journalistic comments on the "battle" at the WHO, see Palca (1991), *New Scientist* (1992), Brown and Patel (1992), and Hornblower (1993).

29. In 1991, the budget fell for the first time from its peak of US$255.5 million to $236.8 million. Although the 1991 figure was still substantially higher than the pre-1990 levels, in effect it represented a steep decline because during the 1980s the number of countries among which it had to be distributed had risen from five to 114 (WHO 1992a).

30. Interview with author, August 17, 1992.

31. Ibid.

32. Author's fieldnotes, December 2, 1992. I am tremendously indebted to Priscilla Alexander, who was at this time the GPA's expert on prostitution and HIV/AIDS. She made it possible for me to come to this important meeting, discussed the issues and participants with me, and allowed me to read her own notes from this and other meetings of the working group. The analysis here, particularly whatever mistakes I may have made or misunderstandings I may have had, is in no way her responsibility, however.

33. Interviews with author, July 13, 1992, and December 1, 1992.

34. Interview with author, November 2, 1992.

35. Interview with author, November 3, 1992.

36. Interview with author, August 10, 1992.

37. Interview with author, November 2, 1992.

38. Interview with author, November 27, 1992.

4. "High-Frequency Transmitters" and Invisible Men

1. Some of the nurses at the clinics I visited during my fieldwork referred to us as "*akina* Ngugi." *Akina* literally means "of the family of" but is colloquially used to refer to a group of people who are the followers or slightly subordinated friends of someone more well known. I was a bit stunned at being referred to as "*akina* Ngugi," but the comment made me realize how closely nurses associated me with this research group.

2. Plummer et al. wrote the chapter on prostitution (1998). Others contributed chapters on chancroid (Ronald and Albritton 1998), pregnancy (Watts and Brunham 1998), infertility (Cates and Brunham 1998), and managing STDs in "developing countries" (de Cock and Katabira 1998).

3. One of their most interesting and most explicitly political articles analyzed the effects of the government's attempt to introduce fees for formerly free STD examinations at Casino. Moses et al. (1992) demonstrated just how negatively the new policy affected attendance and, therefore, STD and HIV prevention.

4. I have been especially influenced by Mary Louise Pratt (1992), Londa Schiebinger (1993), Evelynn Hammonds (1997), Ann L. Stoler (1989a, 1989b, 1991), and Sandra Harding (1993), all of whom bring feminist and anti-racist critiques of science and medicine together to broaden our understanding of how claims to objectivity are used to create, legitimize, and naturalize a specific sexual, race, class, and gender hierarchy. Of course, radical AIDS researchers have done enormously important work on race, class, sexuality, and gender in the making of AIDS knowledge. See especially Donna Haraway (1991), Paula Treichler (1988a, 1988b, and 1999), Randall Packard (1989), Stephen Epstein (1996), and Sander Gilman (1988). Much of this work draws on Foucault's critique of Western European medical and sexual discourses (1977 and 1997) and Edward Said's analysis of the textual production of imperial rule in the Middle East (1978).

5. In the group's first article, they hinted at the model that was to come. They reported on the accuracy of clinical diagnoses of chancroid and the effectiveness of antibiotic treatments. They studied "the first five patients with genital ulcers attending the clinic [Casino] during one morning each week" over three months. They found that 95 of 97 of the patients were men.

Forty-four of the men were married, but only eight lived with their wives in Nairobi. Many of the men had migrated to Nairobi and were physically separated from their wives in the villages for long periods of time. The source of infection was usually reported to be prostitutes, and only two men had had sexual contact with their wives. Most of the contacts occurred in Nairobi (Nsanze et al. 1981, 380).

They do not discuss the situations of the two women who had genital-ulcer disease. In the discussion section of the article, they report that "the patients were mainly of low socio-economic class and acquired their disease from prostitutes" (380).

6. See, for example, Walkowitz (1980), Brandt (1987), Levine (1999), Vaughan (1991), Dawson (1983 and 1988), and Martens (2001).

7. The term "vector" is an epidemiological term referring to an organism that transmits or carries a pathogen from one host to another host. Usually the vector itself does not get ill. The best example of a vector is the anopheles mosquito, which carries the malaria pathogen from one human to another. I marvel at the application of this term to describe the human epidemiology of HIV; HIV is only spread by direct or (very rarely now) indirect human contact; there is no intermediate "carrier" who remains symptom free, at least as far as we know. Moreover, to designate one group of people as "vectors" is to make their own infections relevant only as they lead to the infection of another group or individual, not as a tragedy in themselves. It is interesting that here men who visit prostitutes, not prostitutes themselves, are referred to as vectors of HIV.

8. It is interesting that this article actually suggested that the spread of STDs in Nairobi was not necessarily different from that occurring elsewhere. The authors linked the main characteristic of Nairobi's heterosexual organization—the large numbers of "young men who were either unmarried or physically separated from their wives"—to a presumably more general "situation that occurs during wartime" (Nsanze et al. 1981, 380). This avenue of inquiry is soon dropped, however, in favor of statements about how different heterosexuality, prostitution, and STD transmission in Africa is from such relations in European and North American countries.

9. The term "core group" came eventually to replace "reservoir" (which had replaced "pool") in the writings of Plummer's team. It is certainly a less immediately negative, stigmatizing, and gendered term. The team did not really adopt "core group" wholesale until the late 1990s, however; the "reservoir" metaphor had already been taken up and used in many reports. Simply because there is so much more research on AIDS now, the influence of the Plummer group's work has probably decreased.

10. In the last chapter, we saw how Jonathan Mann's efforts to defuse international hostilities over how AIDS started included propagating the "pattern" paradigm based, apparently, on an objective assessment of epidemiological "difference." The most important article to come out after the 1986

report announcing the arrival of HTLV-III in Nairobi was a review Plummer and co-authors published in *Science* in 1988. "AIDS: An International Perspective" described AIDS as "a worldwide health problem that requires a global approach for control" on the one hand and as a collection of seemingly unlinked regional "patterns" of spread on the other (Piot et al. 1988). The most important of these regional patterns were, of course, the "African" and the "Western" patterns. This article based its conceptualization of the former on the model and data described by Plummer's Nairobi group.

11. Cameron et al. (1989) assert:

> Men who have sexual intercourse with these women have very high risk of exposure to HIV-1; such men also have a high risk of acquiring another STD concomitantly and could be identified on presentation for treatment of that STD. The incubation periods of non-HIV STDs are much shorter than the time of development of antibody to HIV-1, so serial serology of a group of men who acquired an STD from this group of women would allow measurement of the rate of HIV-1 transmission. (404)

12. Of 186 articles indexed in the Medline database under Plummer as author, 59 are categorized under the subject heading "prostitution" and 21 under the subject headings "pregnancy," "maternal," or "mothers." Of these 80 articles, only 2 fit into both subject categories.

13. Some of the most important of these studies are Temmerman et al. (1990), Temmerman and Ryder (1991), Datta et al. (1994), and Jenniskens et al. (1995).

14. There is a clear historical legacy of doing this, as well. In their 1972 article on the determinants of gonorrhea incidence in Kenya, Verhagen and Gemert conclude from their data that prostitutes are the cause of high rates of venereal disease in Nairobi. The basis for this conclusion, however, is that one-third of the gonorrhea-infected women in their sample reported being prostitutes. One-third is no small proportion, of course. The fact that fully two-thirds of urban women with the infection were not prostitutes is simply not accounted for in the model, however. These authors imply that the women's reports cannot be trusted.

15. See Delacoste and Alexander (1987), de Zalduondo (1991), Pheterson (1989), Alexander (1996), and Gorna (1996).

16. Several of these groups have been heralded as examples of successful "grassroots" HIV-prevention projects (Doyal 1994).

17. For a revealing contrast, see Michelle Lewis Renaud's (1997) description of Senegalese sex workers' attempts to get condoms from public health workers in Dakar.

18. The dangers of binary thinking in the context of HIV have been discussed by activists and scholars since the discovery of AIDS. Alonso and Koreck

(1989), Treichler (1988a and 1988b), Patton (1990, 1992, and 1994), Hollibaugh (1999 and 2000), and Farmer (1992) are among the many who have shown us how oppositions between heterosexual and homosexual, lesbian and gay, Haitian or African and American, drug "abuser" and everyone else, and black and white have produced false categories of people who are "at risk." Such categories encourage a dangerous denial among people who do not identify with the identity that is supposedly at risk and an equally dangerous stigmatization of those who do so identify.

19. In their study of women STD patients, Bradley et al. (1992) offer evidence that suggests that research into mothers' sexual behaviors might challenge such an assumption. They found that while significantly fewer married women with STDs than married male patients reported having "extramarital sex," 7 percent of the former, including an unspecified number of pregnant women, had slept with someone other than their husbands within the previous three months. Forty-three percent of unmarried women with STDs, most of whom were also pregnant and did not identify as sex workers, reported having had at least two sexual partners in that period. There is no consideration of these findings in the analysis offered by this or other articles authored by the research team.

20. Bob Rodriguez (1997) has demonstrated that even after women had been "added" to the biomedical understanding of HIV, their bodies and experiences remained marginal to the production of further knowledge about HIV.

21. As Cindy Patton (1990) has argued, there was also a return migration of racist discourse as researchers began to see AIDS in African-American communities as an expression of the "African AIDS" they had previously constructed.

22. This discussion of the importance of metaphor in science is influenced particularly by Emily Martin's well-known essay "The Sperm and the Egg" (1996). Martin demonstrates how U.S. medical textbooks present the story of fertilization to medical students by describing sperm as a man, or group of men, actively pursuing the cherished object, the egg, or woman. The egg is placid, static, and passive. Martin argues that because they are translated as "common sense," the heavily gendered metaphors of heterosexual dating reproduce and support sexist gynecological and obstetric research and practices and make it very difficult for patients or practitioners to challenge such practices. Many others have discussed the power of scientific metaphors, particularly in the age of AIDS. See, for example, Longino (1990), Haraway (1991), Sontag (1989), Gilman (1988), Stepan and Gilman (1991), Martin (1994), Stepan (1982 and 1996), and Treichler (1999).

23. Some of the most important or influential discussions of illness metaphors can be found in Sontag (1989), Gilman (1988), Martin (1994 and 1996), and Kleinman (1980). Sontag's view differs from that of many others and from my own, however. She argues that as diseases become better known

scientifically, the discourse surrounding them becomes less metaphorical (and stigmatizing) and more "scientific." I align myself with the more critical and cynical view that scientific language is no less metaphorical than any other language (although its metaphors have more legitimacy and authority and are less democratically produced than those of poetry, fiction, feminist theory, and so on). Scientific language does not become less metaphorical as it "progresses," although the metaphors may change.

24. Although Treichler invented the now-famous phrase "epidemic of signification," many AIDS activists and scholars before and since have analyzed the meanings and effects produced by efforts to define and contain the new disease. See especially Crimp (1988), Watney (1989a and 1989b), Gilman (1988), Sontag (1989), Martin (1996), Haraway (1991), Chirimuuta and Chirimuuta (1989), and Patton (1990 and 1992).

25. This harboring metaphor is reminiscent of the posters used by the U.S. and British armies during World War II and since to warn soldiers of the dangers of venereal disease. Historian Alan Brandt (1987) describes how U.S. and European prostitutes were represented as women who look fine on the outside but are really serving as harborers of the diseases that will destroy our military might. But in the U.S. military, according to Brandt, the focus was not on changing or getting rid of the prostitutes. Instead the focus was on that which the military believed it could control: male sexuality.

26. For very similar language in another article by the team, see Kreiss et al. (1994).

27. It is interesting that this is something of a reversal of the relationship between the sperm and the egg described by Emily Martin (1996). It also contrasts with the representation of men as the migratory, mobile, moving, active ones in the high-frequency transmission model articulated by Plummer and his team.

28. According to the U.S. Public Health Service's National Pediatric and Family HIV Resource Center (1999), the average risk of HIV transmission from a man to a woman is 0.05 to 0.15 percent per sexual contact. The risk per sexual contact from woman to man is 0.03 to 0.09 percent. The authors do not state whether these are global or national averages.

29. Luise White's history of sexuality in colonial Nairobi is based on the oral histories she was able to collect from women who had lived and worked in the Pumwani area from the 1920s until after World War II. Based on these amazing, and all-too-rarely recorded, histories, White argues that sex work was just one of many entrepreneurial strategies in which early female migrants to Nairobi engaged. Their main strategy was to build their own homes and become landladies. A significant number of them were successful until the 1940s because the colonial government's interests in providing cheap lodging to bachelor male workers coincided with the women's interests. After the two world wars, urban "reforms" forced the women out of their homes and economic depression pushed more rural women into the

city, increasing competition among and diversifying the economic interests of women. Nevertheless, White argues convincingly that as landladies and domestic and sex workers, Pumwani's early female residents were crucial in the founding of the male working class in Kenya.

30. For an example of a scientific article that does insist on understanding the social contexts of sex work and the everyday lives of sex workers, see Karim et al. (1995). This article on sex workers in South Africa is first and foremost concerned with protecting sex workers (rather than their clients or their clients' wives and babies). It is free of stigmatizing and blaming language. It demonstrates that sex workers, like all women, are vulnerable to male violence. It also reports, however, that sex workers actively negotiate with men over sexual practices.

31. See especially Judith Walkowitz's work (1980) on the efforts of male trade unionists and the British state to control prostitution in the name of public health. She finds that British men constructed a cross-class masculine solidarity to maintain the heterosexual double standard in which only men have permission to be sexually promiscuous; the women with whom they have sex are justly (from the men's perspective) open to social and biological punishment.

32. HIV-vaccine research is enormously expensive in part because it has to overcome daunting microbiological difficulties. The Kenyan project had a setback when one of the apparently uninfected prostitutes tested positive for HIV, casting doubt on their initial discovery that all of the uninfected women had a genetic immunity. A more significant problem has confronted all of those who have tried to develop a vaccine. HIV is apparently not just one virus. We have learned that it is more like a category of many types and subtypes of an unstable and quickly mutating pathogen. Different regions and even different countries within one region have different dominant subtypes. We can expect more subtypes to develop in the future. Genetic immunity to HIV appears to be subtype specific. Researchers are trying to determine if a single vaccine or even a small number of vaccines can stop such a complex and unpredictable virus.

33. The International AIDS Vaccine Initiative (IAVI) based in the United Kingdom was established to cope with just this problem by working independently to collect funds from governments, philanthropists, individuals, and corporations. Along with Oxford University, the IAVI is now overseeing the Nairobi project.

34. For a discussion of the effects of the historical domination by men of scientific "fact-making," see Hubbard (1989).

---

5. "A Husband Can Have a Thousand Girlfriends!"

1. Author's fieldnotes, May 14, 1993.

2. The country's first "cost-sharing" scheme, as the World Bank officially

calls it, was a disaster. After it was introduced, the country's citizens protested with their voices and with their feet, boycotting health care centers and hospitals. The first cost-sharing effort collapsed after about a year (Collins et al. 1996). Stephen Moses of the Plummer STD/AIDS research project described in the last chapter was the lead author of an excellent article documenting the fact that fewer patients came in for STD treatment after cost-sharing started (Moses et al. 1992). This is the only article to come out of the group's twenty-year research project that criticizes both the state and the international donor agencies for their failure to recognize the needs of working-class Kenyans at risk of getting HIV. In late 1993, the government made a second attempt to introduce cost-sharing. When I did my fieldwork at Bestlands, the first cost-sharing attempt had already failed and the second one had yet to begin. Nurses and patients alike, however, were still reeling from the fiasco. The nurses did not know if or when they would be told to collect fees again. They also told me that they believed many women thought they would still have to pay a fee for services and were therefore not coming in for care.

3. Author's fieldnotes, May 8, 1993.

4. Author's fieldnotes, June 17, 1993.

5. Bestlands was neither the largest nor the smallest of the five. The staff and members of the research team described it as "typical" in terms of the practices of its health care workers and of how the STD project was progressing. I cannot judge whether this is true.

6. Grace, the nurse who examines women before giving them birth control, refers patients with what she suspects is an STD to Mary and Wamuuchi in what they called the "STD Room" or "Room 2." If Grace observed a suspicious vaginal discharge or heard complaints of itching, for example, she was supposed to send the woman to the clinical officer for examination. Often the clinical officer was not there, however. In addition, Mary and Wamuuchi had more training in STD diagnosis than did the clinical officer—a result of long years of neglect of STDs by the medical school. Patients were almost always sent directly to the "STD Room," bypassing the clinical officer. The "STD nurses," as the two women have come to be called by the other staff, diagnose the STD among the following possible categories: genital-ulcer disease, nongonococcal urethritis, trichomonas vaginitis/candidiasis, pelvic inflammatory disease, gonorrhea, and syphilis. They then determine the appropriate drug therapy. Next, they make up the packet of drugs, record the diagnosis and treatment given, and give the patient the drugs. In the case of several of these infections, the patient is required to take the treatment in front of the nurses before leaving the health care center. They conclude by telling the patient in either Kikuyu or Kiswahili when to return for follow-up and what the implications of her infection might be.

7. Author's fieldnotes, May 28, 1993.

8. The Bamako Initiative was created in the 1970s as a revolving drug fund from which poor countries could get funds for whatever the WHO defined as "essential" drugs.

9. Personal communication with project staff member, April 1995. I took these comments from a letter written to me in response to an earlier version of this chapter in which I blamed the project for being unsustainable and knowingly engineering a dependency in the health care center.

10. Author's fieldnotes, June 10, 1993. The staff made it clear to me that having the drugs had fundamentally affected their ability to do their job of delivering care to women patients. Before the project started, the nurses had to refer patients to several different health care centers around the city to get the various tests (blood and urine) the center needed in order to know how to treat them. As one nurse told me, the center lost patients in that process: "These working-class women might tell you, 'Tomorrow, I may not get permission [to take time from my job] so tell me the results now.'" Now, with the project, "these ones we can tell them to come in the afternoon [of the same day]" rather than send them away and never see them again (author's fieldnotes, June 10, 1993). It is difficult to overestimate the appreciation the staff felt for this change, which was made possible solely by the presence of a syphilis-screening kit, STD drugs, and several training sessions.

11. Author's fieldnotes, June 2, 1993.

12. Author's fieldnotes, June 3, 1993.

13. The Luo and the Kikuyu are the two largest of Kenya's seventeen ethnic groups. Most of the nurses at Bestlands were Kikuyu. Although many Kenyans insist on the truth of mostly negative stereotypes of each ethnic group (except their own), Bestlands' nurses rarely commented to me on any patient's ethnic group. Officially, there is no "tribalism" in Kenya; one is not supposed to ask what tribe another comes from. It is interesting, however, that there is still a "tribe" category in the register where information about new patients is recorded and kept. As I looked through this book I noticed that nurses sometimes recorded a tribe and sometimes did not. I could not discover a pattern, and the nurses were unwilling to discuss it at all.

14. Author's fieldnotes, July 3, 1993.

15. I have here adopted terms popular in the United States to describe class positions. These terms are perhaps not very appropriate in a country that many would argue hardly has a "middle class" at all. It is not, however, clear to me what alternative terminology I could use to indicate the very important and significant differences of wealth and future life chances that exist between these nurses. The Kenyan civil service in general is marked by enormous class inequality; top civil servants are among the ruling elite, while some nurses and many secretaries and clerks can be part of Kenya's

enormous "working poor" majority. The nurses are working people who are neither of the ruling class nor among the poor.

16. Author's fieldnotes, June 10, 1993.

17. Author's fieldnotes, May 27, 1993.

18. Author's fieldnotes, May 29, 1993.

19. Author's fieldnotes, May 8, 1993.

20. There is a marked similarity between this construction of class difference in sexual and reproductive power and that described by Chandra Talpade Mohanty (1991) in her critical analysis of writings by "Western" women on Third World women. The construction is also not unlike those described by Judith Walkowitz (1980) in her study of British middle-class white women's struggles to gain state power by representing working-class and immigrant women as morally inferior and in need of "maternalist" assistance. See also Gordon (1988) and Koven and Michel (1993) for similar discussions of maternalist politics in the United States.

21. Author's fieldnotes, June 7, 1993.

22. Author's fieldnotes, June 12, 1993.

23. In their early discussions of stratification among prostitutes, they did find significant differences in sexual practices and in the prevalence of HIV and other STDs (Plummer et al. 1983). They did not pursue this line of inquiry after the end of the 1980s, however, and never investigated other kinds of class differences among women (or men).

24. In fact, the nurses did not like giving birth control of any kind to women who had not yet had a "successful" pregnancy (that is, one that produced a live baby). Unmarried women who had had several pregnancies could get birth control. Sexually active unmarried women (and even married women) who had not yet delivered a baby could not get birth control. I understood the nurses to be following, if not explicit national policy, widespread norms about who should get birth control. There is a strong current of thought in Kenya, shared apparently by the president (and criticized by many of the nurses I met), that if they are allowed to have birth control, unmarried women will have more sex. Medical practitioners in Kenya estimate that almost 200,000 illegal abortions took place in 1993 and that at least one-third of all maternal deaths result from botched abortions. Doctors working at the country's main public hospital in Nairobi report that on average they see 40 women every day who have suffered complications from illegal abortions (Brockman 1997). It is very likely that the majority of these women are young and unmarried. Needless to say, this suggests that unmarried women are having sex despite the fact that they cannot easily get birth control. Public discussions about the problem of abortion-related deaths in Kenya began in 2002. These continuing discussions suggest that positive policy changes in this area may be on the horizon (Okoko 2002; Kiragu 2003).

25. Author's fieldnotes, May 17, 1993.

26. Ibid.

27. Author's fieldnotes, July 1, 1993.

28. Author's fieldnotes, July 5, 1993.

29. Author's fieldnotes, May 20, 1993.

6. Drugs for Whom?

1. That is, data that provides results that are as likely as possible to be explained *only* by the experimental intervention—here, the administration of AZT.

2. That this antiretroviral drug decreased the amount of HIV in an infected person's blood and helped some patients fight off opportunistic diseases had been celebrated by scientists and people with HIV alike since its discovery at the end of the 1980s. When the U.S. Food and Drug Administration (FDA) approved it for AIDS treatment, many believed a cure was in sight. By 1994, however, HIV-positive Americans and their doctors had discovered that AZT was a fairly weak weapon against the virus when taken alone, had severe side effects, and cost a great deal of money (Manos, Negron, and Horn 2001, 52). Some U.S. scientists were not ready to give up on AZT, however. Connor et al. wanted to know if AZT could be used to prevent HIV transmission in the first place. They hypothesized that if the drug even temporarily reduced the amount of virus in the blood and strengthened the immune system, the virus might be unable to pass from an HIV-positive pregnant woman to her fetus and might thereby prevent the infant-to-be from becoming infected.

3. The campaign in New York actually began in 1993, before scientists had any way to prevent mother-to-child transmission or to distinguish between newborns actually infected with HIV and newborns who had their mothers' antibodies to the virus but not the virus itself. When mothers do not breastfeed, the majority of babies born with HIV antibodies do not actually become HIV positive even if their mothers have not received AZT. I have elsewhere analyzed how anti-gay rhetoric was used by the mainstream New York media to legitimate demands that "at risk" (a code term in this case for poor and African-American or Latina) mothers and their babies be tested for HIV and, if positive, reported to the state (Booth 2000).

4. "Standard" care is theoretically different from "mandatory" treatment. Patients can refuse standard care. In practice, however, patients, particularly those who are poor and pregnant, are frequently not informed that they can do so.

5. It is difficult, by contrast, to find statistics or even estimates of the prevalence of HIV among pregnant women in the United States. Although the overall rate of infection among women of childbearing age (pregnant or not) in the United States is less than 0.1 percent, there is a great deal of variation by state and city. New York, Florida, and New Jersey, for example,

have rates of around 0.5 percent or higher (Abercrombie and Booth 1997). Seventy-eight percent of infections in U.S. women are in African-American women and Latinas (U.S. Public Health Service, National Pediatric and Family HIV Resource Center 1999). Although the United States rarely analyzes the socioeconomic distribution of infection, it is clear from many small studies that, especially among women, HIV infection has mostly affected the poor (Birn, Santelli, and Burwell 1994).

6. Researchers estimate that 70 percent of mother-to-child infections occur during labor or delivery. The other 30 percent occur either earlier in the pregnancy or during breastfeeding. Researchers are unsure what the additional risk from breastfeeding is. Testing technology cannot yet tell us precisely when during pregnancy, labor, or delivery a child becomes infected.

7. The UN moved its lead AIDS group from the WHO to the offices of the UN Development Programme in 1994. While I was doing research at the WHO (two years earlier), there were rumors that this was going to happen and that the WHO's Global Programme on AIDS would be gutted. According to officials, the UN made the move in order to make more clear its understanding that HIV/AIDS had become a "development" issue and to make the office, and the leadership, more open to input from other UN organizations. Some of my interviewees suggested, however, that they thought the move was a (negative) reaction to the changes in policy introduced by Director-General Hiroshi Nakajima of the WHO and by Michael Merson, the head of the GPA.

8. In the 076 study, women in the experimental group were put on AZT at or before thirty-four weeks' gestation (Connor et al. 1994).

9. Marshall (1998a, 1998b) mentions two studies of mother-to-child transmission taking place in Kenya. One NIH-funded study, which Marshall states is finished, compared the effects of bottlefeeding infants of HIV-positive women for three months with the effects of breastfeeding among 450 women. The other was funded by the European Community and examined the effectiveness of "vaginal lavage" (a sort of disinfecting of the birth canal) of 1,000 women just before delivery. Marshall refers to this one as "on-going." He does not indicate whether AZT or any other antiretroviral drug was used or whether the sponsors had ever planned to include a drug in either trial.

10. Personal communication, March 24, 2002. According to de Cock, Kenya hosted only a study of the effects of substituting formula for breast milk among HIV-infected pregnant women. There are also questions about the ethics of comparing formula with breast milk when it is known already that breastfeeding results in HIV infection in a significant proportion of infants born to HIV-positive women.

11. There have recently been debates over nevirapine as well. HIVNET 012 was a trial conducted jointly by Johns Hopkins University and Makerere University in Kampala, Uganda. The trial of oral nevirapine showed that

treatment reduced transmission significantly. But a recent U.S. report obliquely implies that there are some problems:

> An examination of the data to support an extension of the indication for the use of NVP [nevirapine] to include prevention of MTCT [mother-to-child transmission] was recently begun. Although no evidence has been found that the conclusions of HIVNET 012 are invalid or that any trial participants were placed at an increased risk of harm, certain aspects of the collection of the primary data may not conform to FDA regulatory requirements. (NIAID and NIH 2002)

Immediately after issuing this cryptic report, however, the WHO and UNAIDS came out with a joint statement supporting the results of HIVNET 012 and the use of oral NVP to mothers at onset of labor and to newborns within seventy-two hours of birth (UNAIDS and WHO 2002).

12. Despite the still relatively high cost (Burdon 1998).

13. On its excellent Web site, the TAC describes its strategies:

- Promote treatment awareness and treatment literacy among all people.
- Campaign for AZT and Nevirapine for pregnant women to prevent mother-to-child transmissions.
- Campaign against profiteering by drug companies and other bodies.
- Build a mass TAC membership.
- Build networks and alliances with unions, employers, religious bodies, women and youth organisations, lesbian and gay organisations and other interested sections of the community.
- Maintain TAC visibility through posters, pamphlets, meetings, street activism and letter writing. Target pharmaceutical companies to lower the costs of all HIV/AIDS medications and maintain pressure on the government to fulfill its HIV/AIDS obligations. (Available online at <http://www.tac.org.za>. Accessed September 12, 2002.)

14. Such a strategy—save the baby first and regardless—is, of course, not applied only to African women. For many women in the United States—mostly poor, mostly African-American or Latina—AZT to protect their babies is the only drug they can get (Abercrombie and Booth 1997; Booth 2000).

15. Aside from some desultory criticisms of the U.S. government and the pharmaceutical companies, the WHO has been noticeably silent in the debate. Wilson et al. (1999) explain that although in 1999 the World Health Assembly voted to make the Organization monitor "the consequences of international trade agreements" on public health, the WHO's rules prohibited it from intervening without an explicit invitation from a member country. Wilson et al. point out that this makes the WHO effectively powerless to do anything when poor countries such as South Africa and Kenya are under pressure not to challenge the WTO from the countries that hold the purse strings.

Works Cited

Published Documents

Abercrombie, Priscilla, and Karen M. Booth. 1997. "Prevalence of Human Immunodeficiency Virus Infection and Drug Use in Pregnant Women: A Critical Review of the Literature." *Journal of Women's Health* 6: 163–187.

Afshar, Haleh, ed. 1987. *Women, State, and Ideology: Studies from Africa and Asia.* London: Macmillan.

Agonafer, Mulugeta. 1994. *Contending Theories of Development in the Contemporary International Order/Disorder: Lessons from Kenya and Tanzania.* Lanham, Md.: University Press of America.

Ahluwalia, D. Pal S. 1996. *Post-colonialism and the Politics of Kenya.* New York: Nova Science Publishers.

Alexander, Priscilla. 1996. "Making a Living: Women Who Go Out." In *Women's Experiences with HIV/AIDS: An International Perspective,* edited by Lynellen D. Long and E. Maxine Ankrah. New York: Columbia University Press.

Alonso, Ana Maria, and Maria Teresa Koreck. 1989. "Silences: 'Hispanics,' AIDS, and Sexual Practices." *Differences* 1, no. 1: 101–124.

Angell, Marcia. 1997. "The Ethics of Clinical Research in the Third World." *New England Journal of Medicine* 337, no. 12: 847–849.

Arya, O. P., and F. J. Bennett. 1967. "Venereal Disease in an Elite Group (University Students) in East Africa." *British Journal of Venereal Disease* 43: 275–279.

Aubrey, Lisa. 1997. *The Politics of Development Cooperation: NGOs, Gender and Partnership in Kenya.* London: Routledge.

Baleta, Adele. 1999. "When Pharmaceutical Wrangles Cast a Wide Net." *The Lancet* 353 (May 15): 1685.

——. 2000. "Questioning of HIV Theory of AIDS Causes Dismay in South Africa." *The Lancet* 355 (April 1): 1167.

Baraza, Richard. 1998. "Kenyan Statutory Body Was Unaware of Study." *British Medical Journal* 316 (February 21): 625.

Barkan, Joel, and Michael Chege. 1989. "Decentralizing the State: District Focus and the Politics of Reallocation in Kenya." *The Journal of Modern African Studies* 27, no. 3: 431–453.

Bates, Robert H. 1989. *Beyond the Miracle of the Market: The Political Economy of Agrarian Development in Kenya.* Cambridge: Cambridge University Press.

Baylies, Carolyn, and Janet Bujra. 1995. "Discourses of Power and Empowerment in the Fight against HIV/AIDS in Africa." In *AIDS: Safety, Sexuality and Risk,* edited by Peter Aggleton, Peter Davies, and Graham Hurt. London: Taylor & Francis.

Baylies, Carolyn, Janet Bujra, and the Gender and AIDS Group, eds. 2000. *AIDS, Sexuality and Gender in Africa: Collective Strategies and Struggles in Tanzania and Zambia.* London: Routledge.

Beck, Ann. 1981. *Medicine, Tradition, and Development in Kenya and Tanzania, 1920–1970.* Waltham, Mass.: Crossroads.

Benatar, Solomon R., and Peter A. Singer. 2000. "A New Look at International Research Ethics." *British Medical Journal* 321 (September 30): 824–826.

Berman, Bruce J., and John Lonsdale. 1992. *Unhappy Valley: Conflict in Kenya and Africa.* London: James Currey.

Bhabha, Homi. 1984. "Of Mimicry and Man: The Ambivalence of Colonial Discourse." *October* 28 (Spring): 125–133.

Birn, Anne-Emanuelle, John Santelli, and LaWanda G. Burwell. 1994. "Pediatric AIDS in the United States: Epidemiological Reality versus Government Policy." In *AIDS: The Politics of Survival,* edited by Nancy Krieger and Glen Margo. Amityville, N.Y.: Baywood Publishing Co.

Bloom, Barry. 1998. "The Highest Attainable Standard: Ethical Issues in AIDS Vaccines." *Science* 279: 186–188.

Booker, Salih, and William Minter. 2001. "Global Apartheid." *The Nation,* July 9.

Booth, Karen M. 1995. "Technical difficulties: AIDS and the problem of women in Nairobi, Kenya." Ph.D. diss., University of Wisconsin–Madison.

——. 1998. "National Mother/Global Whore: Femocrats and the Politics of AIDS at the World Health Organization." *Feminist Studies* 24: 115–139.

——. 2000. "'Just Testing': Race, Sex, and Blame in New York's 'Baby AIDS' Debate." *Gender & Society* 14 (October): 644–661.

Brandt, Allen. 1987. *No Magic Bullet: A Social History of Venereal Disease in the United States since 1880.* New York: Oxford University Press.

Brilliant, Lawrence B. 1985. *The Management of Smallpox Eradication in India.* Ann Arbor: University of Michigan Press.

Brockman, Norbert. 1997. "Kenya." In *The International Encyclopedia of Sexuality, Volumes 1–3,* edited by Robert T. Francoeur. Available online at <http://www2.rz.hu-berlin.de/sexology/GESUND/ARCHIV/IES>. Accessed March 16, 2003.

Brown, Phyllida, and Tara Patel. 1992. "Mud Flies in Battle for the WHO." *New Scientist* 19, no. 26 (December): 4.

Bujra, Janet, and Carolyn Baylies. 2000. "Responses to the AIDS Epidemic in Tanzania and Zambia." In *AIDS, Sexuality and Gender in Africa*, edited by Baylies, Bujra, and the Gender and AIDS Group.

———. 2001. "Africa: Targeting Men for a Change to Prevent AIDS." *Women's International Network News* 27, no. 1: 18.

Burawoy, Michael. 2000a. "Introduction: Reaching for the Global." In *Global Ethnography: Forces, Connections, and Imaginations in a Postmodern World*, edited by Michael Burawoy, Joseph A. Blum, Sheba George, Zsuzsa Gille, Teresa Gowan, Lynne Haney, Maren Klawiter, Steven H. Lopez, Seán Ó Riain, and Millie Thayer. Berkeley: University of California Press.

———. 2000b. "Grounding Globalization." In *Global Ethnography: Forces, Connections, and Imaginations in a Postmodern World*, edited by Michael Burawoy, Joseph A. Blum, Sheba George, Zsuzsa Gille, Teresa Gowan, Lynne Haney, Maren Klawiter, Steven H. Lopez, Seán O Riain, and Millie Thayer. Berkeley: University of California Press.

Burdon, Justin. 1998. "Zidovudine Is Too Expensive for Developing Countries." *British Medical Journal* 316 (February 21): 625.

Buvé, Anne, Kizito Bishikwabo-Nsarhaza, and Gladys Mutangadura. 2002. "The Spread and Effect of HIV-1 Infection in Sub-Saharan Africa." *The Lancet* 359, no. 9322: 2011–2017.

Bwayo, J. J., A. N. Mutere, A. M. Omari, J. Kreiss, W. Jaoko, C. Sekkade-Kigondu, and F. A. Plummer. 1991. "Long Distance Truck Drivers. 2: Knowledge and Attitudes Concerning Sexually Transmitted Diseases and Sexual Behaviour." *East African Medical Journal* 68, no. 9: 714–719.

Bwayo, J. J., A. M. Omari, A. N. Mutere, W. Jaoko, C. Sekkade-Kigondu, J. Kreiss, and F. A. Plummer. 1991. "Long Distance Truck-Drivers: 1. Prevalence of Sexually Transmitted Diseases (STDs)." *East African Medical Journal* 68, no. 6: 425–429.

Caldwell, John C., and Pat Caldwell. 1993. "The Nature and Limits of the Sub-Saharan African AIDS Epidemic: Evidence from Geographic and Other Patterns." *Population and Development Review* 19, no. 4: 817–848.

Cameron, D. W., J. N. Simonsen, L. J. D'Costa, A. R. Ronald, G. M. Maitha, M. N. Gakinya, M. Cheang, J. O. Ndinya-Achola, P. Piot, R. C. Brunham, and F. A. Plummer. 1989. "Female to Male Transmission of Human Immunodeficiency Virus Type 1: Risk Factors for Seroconversion in Men." *The Lancet* 2 (August 19): 403–408.

Carovano, Kathryn. 1991. "More than Mothers or Whores: Redefining the AIDS Prevention Needs of Women." *International Journal of Health Services* 21, no. 1: 131–142.

Cates, Willard, Jr., and Robert C. Brunham. 1998. "Sexually Transmitted Diseases and Infertility." In *Sexually Transmitted Diseases*, 3d ed., edited by Holmes, Sparling, and Wasserheit.

CDC (Centers for Disease Control and Prevention). 1998. "Administration of Zidovudine during Late Pregnancy and Delivery to Prevent Perinatal HIV

Transmission—Thailand, 1996–1998." *Morbidity and Mortality Weekly Report* 47, no. 8: 151–154.

Chase, Mary. 1953. *Harvey, a Play.* New York: Oxford University Press.

Chirimuuta, Richard, and Roseline Chirimuuta. 1989. *AIDS, Africa, and Racism.* London: Free Association Books.

Collins, David H., Jonathan D. Quick, Stephen N. Musau, and Daniel L. Kraushaar. 1996. *Health Financing Reform in Kenya: The Fall and Rise of Cost Sharing, 1989–94.* Boston: Management Sciences for Health.

Comaroff, Jean. 1993. "The Diseased Heart of Africa: Medicine, Colonialism, and the Black Body." In *Knowledge, Power and Practice,* edited by Shirley Lindenbaum and Margaret Lock. Berkeley: University of California Press.

Connor, Edward M., et al. 1994. "Reduction of Maternal-Infant Transmission of Human Immunodeficiency Virus Type 1 with Zidovudine Treatment." *The New England Journal of Medicine* 331, no. 18: 1173–1180.

Cooper, Frederick. 1983. "Urban Space, Industrial Time, and Wage Labor in Africa." In *Struggle for the City: Migrant Labor, Capital, and the State in Urban Africa,* edited by Frederick Cooper. Beverly Hills, Calif.: Sage.

Crimp, Douglas. 1988. "AIDS: Cultural Analysis/Cultural Activism." In *AIDS: Cultural Analysis/Cultural Activism,* edited by Douglas Crimp. Cambridge, Mass.: MIT Press.

Curtin, Philip D. 1992. "Medical Knowledge and Urban Planning in Colonial Tropical Africa." In *The Social Basis of Health and Healing in Africa,* edited by Steven Feierman and John M. Janzen. Berkeley: University of California Press.

———. 1998. *Disease and Empire: The Health of European Troops in the Conquest of Africa.* Cambridge: Cambridge University Press.

Datta, P., J. E. Embree, J. K. Kreiss, J. O. Ndinya-Achola, M. Braddick, and M. Temmerman. 1994. "Mother-to-Child Transmission of Human Immunodeficiency Virus Type 1." *Journal of Infectious Diseases* 170, no. 5: 1134–1140.

Davis, Paula Jean. 2000. "On the Sexuality of 'Town Women' in Kampala." *Africa Today* 47, no. 3/4: 28–60.

Dawson, Marc H. 1983. "Socio-economic and epidemiological change in Kenya: 1880–1925." Ph.D. diss., University of Wisconsin.

———. 1988. "AIDS in Africa: Historical Roots." In *AIDS in Africa: The Social and Policy Impact,* edited by Norman Miller and R. C. Rockwell. Lewiston, N.Y.: Edwin Mellon Press.

D'Costa, L. J., F. A. Plummer, I. Bowmer, L. Fransen, P. Piot, A. R. Ronald, and H. Nsanze. 1985. "Prostitutes Are a Major Reservoir of Sexually Transmitted Diseases in Nairobi, Kenya." *Sexually Transmitted Diseases* 12, no. 2: 64–67.

de Cock, K. M., M. G. Fowler, E. Mercier, I. de Vincenzi, J. Saba, E. Hoff, D. J. Alnwick, M. Rogers, and N. Shaffer. 2000. "Prevention of Mother-to-Child HIV Transmission in Resource-Poor Countries: Translating Research into Policy and Practice." *Journal of the American Medical Association* 283, no. 9: 1175–1182.

de Cock, Kevin M., and Elly T. Katabira. 1998. "Approach to Management of HIV/AIDS in Developing Countries." In *Sexually Transmitted Diseases*, 3d ed., edited by Holmes, Sparling, and Wasserheit.

Delacoste, Frederique, and Priscilla Alexander. 1987. *Sex Work: Writings by Women in the Sex Industry.* Pittsburgh: Cleis.

des Jarlais, Don C. 1998. Letter. *Science* 279 (March 6): 1431.

Doyal, Lesley. 1994. *AIDS: Setting a Feminist Agenda.* London: Taylor and Francis.

Edi-Osagie, E. C., and N. E. Edi-Osagie. 1998. "Ethics and International Research: Placebo Trials Are Unethical for Established, Untested Treatments." *British Medical Journal* 316, no. 7131: 625–626.

Ehrhardt, Anke A. 1996. "Sexual Behavior among Heterosexuals." In *AIDS in the World II*, edited by Jonathan Mann and Daniel Tarantola. Oxford: Oxford University Press.

Epstein, Steven. 1996. *Impure Science: AIDS, Activism, and the Politics of Knowledge.* Berkeley: University of California Press.

Farmer, Paul. 1992. *AIDS and Accusation: Haiti and the Geography of Blame.* Berkeley: University of California Press.

Fausto-Sterling, Anne. 1995. "Gender, Race, and Nation: The Comparative Anatomy of 'Hottentot' Women in Europe." In *Deviant Bodies*, edited by Jennifer Terry and Jacqueline Urla. Bloomington: Indiana University Press.

Ford, Michael, and Frank Holmquist. 1988. "The State and Economy in Kenya." *African Economic History* 17: 153–163.

Fortin, Alfred J. 1987. "The Politics of AIDS in Kenya." *Third World Quarterly* 9, no. 3: 906–919.

———. 1990. "AIDS, Development and the Limitations of the African State." In *Action on AIDS: National Policies in Comparative Perspective*, edited by Barbara A. Misztal and David Moss. New York: Greenwood.

Foucault, Michel. 1973. *The Birth of the Clinic: An Archaeology of Medical Perception.* Translated from the French by A. M. Sheridan Smith. New York: Pantheon Books.

———. 1977. *Power/Knowledge: Selected Interviews and Other Writings, 1972–1977.* Edited by Colin Gordon. New York: Pantheon.

Fowke, K. R., N. J. Nagelkerke, J. Kimani, J. N. Simonsen, A. O. Anzala, and J. J. Bwayo. 1996. "Resistance to HIV-1 Infection among Persistently Seronegative Prostitutes in Nairobi." *The Lancet* 348, no. 9038: 1347–1351.

Fraser, Nancy. 1989. *Unruly Practices: Power, Discourse, and Gender in Contemporary Social Theory.* Minneapolis: University of Minnesota Press.

Fuentes, Annette, and Barbara Ehrenreich. 1983. *Women in the Global Factory.* Boston: South End.

Gellman, Barton. 2000. "The Belated Global Response to AIDS in Africa: World Shunned Signs of the Coming Plague." *The Washington Post*, July 5, A1.

Gertzel, Cherry J. 1970. *The Politics of Independent Kenya, 1963–8.* Evanston, Ill.: Northwestern University Press.

Gilman, Sander, L. 1985. *Black Bodies, White Bodies: Toward an Iconography of Female Sexuality.* Chicago: University of Chicago Press.

———. 1988. *Disease and Representation: The Construction of Images of Illness from Madness to AIDS.* Ithaca, N.Y.: Cornell University Press.

Gĩthĩnjĩ, Mwangi wa. 2000. *Ten Millionaires and Ten Million Beggars: A Study of Income Distribution and Development in Kenya.* Aldershot: Ashgate.

Glynn, J., M. Caraël, B. Auvert, M. Kahindo, J. Chege, and R. Musonda. 2001. "Why Do Young Women Have a Much Higher Prevalence of HIV than Young Men? A Study in Kisumu, Kenya and Ndola, Zambia." *AIDS* 15 (S4): S51–S60.

Gordon, April A. 2001. "Population, Urbanization, and AIDS." In *Understanding Contemporary Africa*, 3d ed., edited by April A. Gordon and Donald L. Gordon. Boulder: Lynne Rienner.

Gordon, Linda. 1988. *Heroes of Their Own Lives: The Politics and History of Family Violence, Boston, 1880–1960.* New York: Viking.

Gorna, Robin. 1996. *Vamps, Virgins and Victims: How Can Women Fight AIDS?* London: Cassell.

Greenblatt, R. M., S. A Lukehart, F. A. Plummer, T. C. Quinn, C. W. Critchlow, R. L. Ashley, L. J. D'Costa, J. O. Ndinya-Achola, L. Corey, and A. R. Ronald. 1988. "Genital Ulceration as a Risk Factor for Human Immunodeficiency Virus Infection." *AIDS* 2, no. 1: 47–50.

Gregory, Robert G. 1993. *South Asians in East Africa: An Economic and Social History, 1890–1980.* Boulder: Westview.

Grewal, Inderpal. 1996. *Home and Harem: Nationalism, Imperialism, and the Culture of Travel.* Durham, N.C.: Duke University Press.

Grindle, Merilee Serrill. 1996. *Challenging the State: Crisis and Innovation in Latin America and Africa.* Cambridge: Cambridge University Press.

Gupta, Akhil. 1998. *Postcolonial Developments: Agriculture in the Making of Modern India.* Durham, N.C.: Duke University Press.

Hammond, G. W., M. Slutchuk, J. Scatliff, E. Sherman, J. C. Wilt, and A. R. Ronald. 1980. "Epidemiologic, Clinical, Laboratory, and Therapeutic Features of an Urban Outbreak of Chancroid in North America." *Reviews of Infectious Diseases* 2, no. 6: 867–879.

Hammonds, Evelynn M. 1997. "Seeing AIDS: Race, Gender, and Representation." In *The Gender Politics of HIV/AIDS in Women: Perspectives on the Pandemic in the United States*, edited by Nancy Goldstein and Jennifer L. Manlowe. New York: New York University Press.

Haraway, Donna. 1988. "Situated Knowledges: The Science Question in Feminism and the Privilege of Partial Perspectives." *Feminist Studies* 14 (Fall): 575–599.

———. 1989. *Primate Visions: Gender, Race, and Nature in the World of Modern Science.* New York: Routledge.

———. 1991. "The Politics of Postmodern Bodies: Constitutions of Self in Immune System Discourse." In *Simians, Cyborgs, and Women.* New York: Routledge.

Harding, Sandra G., ed. 1993. *The "Racial" Economy of Science: Toward a Democratic Future.* Bloomington: Indiana University Press.

Hartmann, Betsy. 1995. *Reproductive Rights and Wrongs: The Global Politics of Population Control.* Revised ed. Boston: South End.

Haugerud, Angelique. 1995. *The Culture of Politics in Modern Kenya.* Cambridge: Cambridge University Press.

Himbara, David. 1994. *Kenyan Capitalists, the State, and Development.* Boulder: Lynne Rienner.

Hine, Darlene Clark, ed. 1985. *Black Women in the Nursing Profession: A Documentary History.* New York: Garland.

Hollibaugh, Amber. 1999. "Lesbian Denial and Lesbian Leadership in the AIDS Epidemic: Bravery and Fear in the Construction of a Lesbian Geography of Risk." In *Women Resisting AIDS,* edited by Schneider and Stoller.

———. 2000. "Transmission, Transmission, Where's the Transmission?" In *My Dangerous Desires: A Queer Girl Dreaming Her Way Home.* Durham, N.C.: Duke University Press. Originally published in *Sojourner,* June 1994.

Holmes, King K., ed. 1992. *Sexually Transmitted Diseases.* 2d ed. New York: McGraw.

Holmes, King K., Per-Anders Mardh Sparling, and Judith Wasserheit, eds. 1998. *Sexually Transmitted Diseases.* 3d ed. New York: McGraw-Hill.

Holmquist, Frank, and Michael Ford. 1994. "Kenya: State and Civil Society— The First Year after the Election." *Africa Today* (Fourth Quarter): 5–25.

Holmquist, Frank W., Frederick S. Weaver, and Michael D. Ford. 1994. "The Structural Development of Kenya's Political Economy." *African Studies Review* 37, no. 1: 69–105.

Hoogvelt, Ankie M. 2001. *Globalization and the Postcolonial World: The New Political Economy of Development.* Baltimore: Johns Hopkins University Press.

Hopcraft, M., A. R. Verhagen, S. Ngigi, and A. C. Haga. 1973. "Genital Infections in Developing Countries: Experience in a Family Planning Clinic." *Bulletin of the World Health Organization* 48: 581–586.

Hornblower, Margot. 1993. "Who Leads WHO?" *Time* (January 18): 18.

Huband, Mark. 2001. *The Skull beneath the Skin: Africa after the Cold War.* Boulder: Westview.

Hubbard, Ruth. 1989. "Science, Facts, and Feminism." In *Feminism and Science,* edited by Nancy Tuana. Bloomington: Indiana University Press.

IAVI (International AIDS Vaccine Initiative). 2001. "Women and HIV in Kenya: An interview with Dorothy Mbori-Ngacha." Available online at <http://www.iavi.org/reports/262/women_and_hiv_in_kenya_mbori.htm>. Accessed October 10, 2002.

Jenniskens, Françoise. 1992. *Evaluation of Diagnostic Procedures for Women Attending an STD Referral Clinic in Nairobi, Kenya: Is It Possible in 90 Seconds?* Nairobi: African Medical and Research Foundation.

Jenniskens, F., E. Obwaka, S. Kirisuah, S. Moses, F. M. Yusufali, J. O. Achola, and L. Fransen. 1995. "Syphilis Control in Pregnancy: Decentralization of Screening Facilities to Primary Care." *International Journal of Gynaecology & Obstetrics* 48 (Suppl.): S121–128.

Joffe, Carole. 1986. *The Regulation of Sexuality: Experiences of Family Planning Workers.* Philadelphia: Temple University Press.

Johnson, A., and Marie Laga. 1988. "Heterosexual Transmission of HIV." *AIDS* 2 (Suppl. 1): S49–56.

Johnson, Frederick. 1984. *A Standard Swahili-English Dictionary.* Nairobi: Oxford University Press.

Jones, James H. 1992. *Bad Blood: The Tuskegee Syphilis Experiment.* Revised ed. New York: Free Press.

Kaplan, Caren, Norma Alarcon, and Minoo Moallem, eds. 1999. *Between Woman and Nation: Nationalisms, Transnational Feminisms, and the State.* Durham, N.C.: Duke University Press.

Karim, Quarraisha Abdool, Salim S. Abdool Karim, Kate Soldan, and Martin Zondi. 1995. "Reducing the Risk of HIV Infection among South African Sex Workers: Socioeconomic and Gender Barriers." *American Journal of Public Health* 85, no. 11: 1521–1525.

Kaul, R., F. A. Plummer, J. Kimani, T. Dong, P. Kiama, T. Rostron, E. Njagi, and K. MacDonald. 2000. "HIV-1-Specific Mucosal CD8+ Lymphocyte Responses in the Cervix of HIV-1-Resistant Kenyan Sex Workers." *Journal of Immunology* 164, no. 3: 1602–1611.

Kennedy, Dane Keith. 1987. *Islands of White: Settler Society and Culture in Kenya and Southern Rhodesia, 1890–1939.* Durham, N.C.: Duke University Press.

Kershaw, Greet. 1997. *Mau Mau from Below.* Oxford: James Currey.

Kibukamusoke, J. W. 1965. "Venereal Disease in East Africa." *Transactions of the Royal Society of Tropical Medicine and Hygiene* 59, no. 6: 642–648.

Kiragu, Jane. 2003. "Comment. Let's Not Simplify the Abortion Debate." *The Nation* (Kenya), March 15. Available online at <http://allafrica.com/stories/200303150072.html>. Accessed March 16, 2003.

Kirmani, Mubina Hassanali, and Dorothy Munyakho. 1996. "The Impact of Structural Adjustment Programs on Women and AIDS." In *Women's Experiences with HIV/AIDS: An International Perspective,* edited by Lynellen D. Long and E. Maxine Ankrah. New York: Columbia University Press.

Kitching, Gavin N. 1980. *Class and Economic Change in Kenya: The Making of an African Petite Bourgeoisie, 1905–1970.* New Haven, Conn.: Yale University Press.

———. 1985. "Politics, Method, and Evidence in the 'Kenya Debate.'" In *Contradictions of Accumulation in Africa,* edited by Henry Bernstein and Bonnie K. Campbell. London: Sage.

Kleinman, Arthur. 1980. *Patients and Healers in the Context of Culture.* Berkeley: University of California Press.

Konotey-Ahulu, F. I. 1987. "AIDS in Africa: Misinformation and Disinformation." *The Lancet* 2, no. 8552: 206–207.

Koven, Seth, and Sonya Michel, eds. 1993. *Mothers of a New World: Maternalist Politics and the Origins of Welfare States.* New York: Routledge.

Kreiss, J. K., R. Coombs, F. Plummer, K. K. Holmes, B. Nikora, W. Cameron, and E. Ngugi. 1989. "Isolation of Human Immunodeficiency Virus from

Genital Ulcers in Nairobi Prostitutes." *Journal of Infectious Diseases* 160, no. 3: 380–384.

Kreiss, J. K., D. Koech, F. A. Plummer, K. K. Holmes, M. Lightfoote, P. Piot, and A. R. Ronald. 1986. "AIDS Virus Infection in Nairobi Prostitutes: Spread of the Epidemic to East Africa." *New England Journal of Medicine* 314, no. 7: 414–418.

Kreiss, J., E. Ngugi, K. Holmes, J. Ndinya-Achola, P. Waiyaki, P. L. Roberts, and I. Ruminjo. 1992. "Efficacy of Nonoxynol 9 Contraceptive Sponge Use in Preventing Heterosexual HIV Transmission." *Journal of the American Medical Association* 268, no. 4: 477–482.

Kreiss, J., D. M. Willerford, M. Hensel, W. Emonyi, F. Plummer, and J. Ndinya-Achola. 1994. "Association between Cervical Inflammation and Cervical Shedding of Human Immunodeficiency Virus." *Journal of Infectious Diseases* 170, no. 6: 1597–1601.

Krotz, Larry (director). 1999. *Searching for Hawa's Secret.* National Film Board of Canada. Distributed by First Run/Icarus Films, Brooklyn, New York.

Kunitz, Stephen J. 1987. "Explanations and Ideologies of Mortality Patterns." *Population and Development Review* 13, no. 3: 379–408.

Kurtz, J. Roger. 1998. *Urban Fears, Urban Obsessions: The Postcolonial Kenyan Novel.* Trenton, N.J.: Africa World.

The Lancet. 1993. "Editorial: Ticket to Dignity beyond a Brick Wall." *The Lancet* 341 (8861): 1625.

Langdon, Steven. 1977. "The State and Capitalism in Kenya." *Review of African Political Economy* 8: 90–98.

Layoun, Mary. 1991. "Telling Spaces: Palestinian Women and the Engendering of National Narratives." In *Nationalisms and Sexualities,* edited by Andrew Parker, Mary Russo, Doris Summer, and Patricia Yeager. New York: Routledge.

———. 2001. *Wedded to the Land? Gender, Boundaries, and Nationalism in Crisis.* Durham, N.C.: Duke University Press.

Levine, Phillippa. 1999. "Modernity, Medicine and Colonialism: The Contagious Diseases Ordinances in Hong Kong and the Straits Settlements." In *Gender, Sexuality and Colonial Modernities,* edited by Antoinette Burton. London: Routledge.

Lewis, Joanna. 2000. *Empire State-Building: War & Welfare in Kenya, 1925–52.* Oxford: James Currey.

Lewis, Neil A. 1999. "U.S. Industry to Drop AIDS Drug Lawsuit against South Africa." *New York Times,* September 10, A3.

Leys, Colin. 1975. *Colonial Economy.* Berkeley: University of California Press.

———. 1994. *African Capitalists in African Development.* Boulder: Lynne Rienner.

Likimani, Muthoni G. 1985. *Passbook Number F.47927: Women and Mau Mau in Kenya.* Basingstoke: Macmillan.

Longino, Helen. 1990. *Science as Social Knowledge.* Princeton, N.J.: Princeton University Press.

Lurie, Peter, and Sidney M. Wolfe. 1997a. "Unethical Trials of Interventions to Reduce Perinatal Transmission of the Human Immunodeficiency Virus in Developing Countries." *New England Journal of Medicine* 337, no. 12: 853–856.

———. 1997b. Letter to the Department of Health and Human Services concerning unethical studies which used placebos on HIV-positive pregnant women in developing countries. (HRG Publication #1430). Website of Public Citizen. Available online at <http://www.citizen.org/publications/release.cfm?ID=6627>. Accessed March 23, 2002.

Lutz, Catherine, and Jane L. Collins. 1993. *Reading National Geographic.* Chicago: University of Chicago Press.

Lyall, T. 1959. "Venereal Disease in Kenya: An Attempt to Assess the Probable Extent of the Problem." Unpublished report to the Ninth Session of the World Health Organization Regional Committee for Africa, Nairobi, September 21–26.

MacDonald, K. S., et al. 2000. "Influence of HLA Supertypes on Susceptibility and Resistance to Human Immunodeficiency Virus." *Journal of Infectious Diseases* 181, no. 5: 1581–1589.

Mann, Jonathan. 1987. "AIDS in Africa." *New Scientist* 26 (March): 40–43.

———. 1988. "AIDS: A Global Report." In *AIDS and Associated Cancers in Africa: 2nd International Symposium,* edited by G. Giraldo, E. Beth-Giraldo, N. Clumeck, M. R. Gharbi, S. K. Kyalwazi, and G. The. Basel: Karger.

Mann, J. M., J. Chin, P. Piot, and T. Quinn. 1988. "The International Epidemiology of AIDS." *Scientific American* 259, no. 4: 82–89.

Mann, Jonathan, and Kathleen Kay. 1991. "Confronting the Pandemic: The World Health Organization's Global Programme on AIDS, 1986–1989." *AIDS* 5 (Suppl. 2): S221–229.

Mann, Jonathan, Daniel J. M. Tarantola, and Thomas W. Netter. 1992. *AIDS in the World.* Cambridge: Harvard University Press.

Manos, George, Leonardo Negron, and Tim Horn. 2001. "Antiviral Drugs." In *Encyclopedia of AIDS,* edited by Raymond A. Smith. New York: Penguin Books.

Marks, Shula. 1994. *Divided Sisterhood: Race, Class, and Gender in the South African Nursing Profession.* New York: St. Martin's.

Marshall, Eliot. 1998a. "AIDS Therapy: Controversial Trial Offers Hopeful Result." *JAMA HIV/AIDS Resource Center.* Available online at <http://www.ama-assn.org/special/hiv/newsline/special/science/1299.htm>. Accessed October 10, 2002.

———. 1998b. "Controversial Trial Offers Hopeful Result." *Science Magazine* 279, no. 5355: 1299.

Martens, Jeremy C. 2001. "'Almost a public calamity': Prostitutes, 'Nurse-boys,' and Attempts to Control Venereal Diseases in Natal, 1886–1890." *South African Historical Journal* 45: 27–52.

Martin, Emily. 1994. *Flexible Bodies: The Role of Immunity in American Culture from the Days of Polio to the Age of AIDS.* Boston: Beacon.

———. 1996. "The Egg and the Sperm: How Science Has Constructed a Romance Based on Stereotypical Male-Female Roles." In *Feminism and Science,* edited by Evelyn Fox Keller and Helen E. Longino. Oxford: Oxford University Press.

Martin, H. L., D. J. Jackson, K. Mandaliya, J. Bwayo, J. P. Rakwar, P. Nyange, and S. Moses. 1994. "Preparation for AIDS Vaccine Evaluation in Mombasa, Kenya." *AIDS Research & Human Retroviruses* 10 (Suppl. 2): S235–237.

Massey, Doreen. 1994. *Space, Place, and Gender.* Cambridge: Polity Press.

Maughan-Brown, David. 1985. *Land, Freedom, and Fiction: History and Ideology in Kenya.* London: Zed Books.

Mbidde, E. K. 1998. "Bioethics and Local Circumstances." *Science* 279 (January 9): 155.

Mbilinyi, Marjorie, and Naomi Kaihula. 2000. "Sinners and Outsiders: The Drama of AIDS in Rungwe." In *AIDS, Sexuality and Gender in Africa: Collective Strategies and Struggles in Tanzania and Zambia,* edited by Carolyn Baylies, Janet Bujra, and the Women and AIDS Group. London: Routledge.

Mburu, F. M. 1981. "Implications of the Ideology and Implementation of Health Policy in a Developing Country." *Social Science and Medicine* 15: 17–24.

———. 1992. "The Social Construction of Health Care in Kenya." In *The Social Basis of Health and Healing in Africa,* edited by Stephen Feierman and John M. Janzen. Berkeley: University of California Press.

Mburu, John. 2000. "Awakenings: Dreams and Delusions of an Incipient Lesbian and Gay Movement in Kenya." In *Different Rainbows,* edited by Peter Drucker. London: Millivres.

McClintock, Anne. 1995. *Imperial Leather: Race, Gender, and Sexuality in the Colonial Conquest.* New York: Routledge.

McIntosh, Kenneth. 1998. "Short (and Shorter) Courses of Zidovudine." *New England Journal of Medicine* 339, no. 20: 1467–1468.

Modleski, Tania. 1992. "Cinema and the Dark Continent: Race and Gender in Popular Film." In *American Feminist Thought at Century's End,* edited by Linda S. Kauffman. Cambridge, Mass.: Blackwell.

Mohanty, Chandra Talpade. 1991. "Under Western Eyes: Feminist Scholarship and Colonial Discourses." In *Third World Women and the Politics of Feminism,* edited by Chandra Talpade Mohanty, Ann Russo, and Lourdes Torres. Bloomington: Indiana University Press.

Monti-Catania, Diane. 1997. "Women, Violence, and HIV/AIDS." In *The Gender Politics of HIV/AIDS in Women: Perspectives on the Pandemic in the United States,* edited by Nancy Goldstein and Jennifer L. Manlowe. New York: New York University Press.

Moses, S., F. Manji, J. E. Bradley, N. J. Nagelkerke, M. A. Malisa, and F. A. Plummer. 1992. "Impact of User Fees on Attendance at a Referral Centre for Sexually Transmitted Diseases." *The Lancet* 340, no. 8817: 463–466.

Moses, S., E. Muia, J. E. Bradley, N. J. Nagelkerke, E. N. Ngugi, E. K. Njeru, and G. Eldridge. 1994. "Sexual Behaviour in Kenya: Implications for Sexually Transmitted Disease Transmission." *Social Science & Medicine* 39, no. 12: 1649–1656.

Moses, S., F. A. Plummer, E. N. Ngugi, N. J. Nagelkerke, A. O. Anzala, and J. O. Ndinya-Achola. 1991. "Controlling HIV in Africa: Effectiveness and Cost of an Intervention in a High-Frequency Transmitter Core Group." *AIDS* 5, no. 4: 407–411.

Moss, G. B., D. Clemetson, L. D'Costa, F. A. Plummer, J. O. Ndinya-Achola, and M. Reilly. 1991. "Association of Cervical Ectopy with Heterosexual Transmission of Human Immunodeficiency Virus." *Journal of Infectious Diseases* 164, no. 3: 588–591.

Mudimbe, V. Y. 1988. *The Invention of Africa: Gnosis, Philosophy, and the Order of Knowledge*. Bloomington: Indiana University Press.

Myers, Steven Lee. 1999. "South Africa and U.S. End Dispute over Drugs." *New York Times*, September 18, A8.

Ndinya-Achola, J. O., A. E. Ghee, A. N. Kihara, M. R. Krone, F. A. Plummer, and L. D. Fisher. 1997. "High HIV Prevalence, Low Condom Use, and Gender Differences in Sexual Behaviour." *International Journal of STD & AIDS* 8, no. 8: 506–514.

Nederveen Pieterse, Jan. 1992. *White on Black: Images of Africa and Blacks in Western Popular Culture*. New Haven, Conn.: Yale University Press.

Nelson, Nici. 1987. "'Selling her kiosk': Kikuyu Notions of Sexuality and Sex for Sale in Mathare Valley, Kenya." In *The Cultural Construction of Sexuality*, edited by Pat Caplan. London: Tavistock.

New Scientist. 1992. "WHO's in Trouble?" 136 (1852/1853): 3.

Ngugi, E. N., F. A. Plummer, J. N. Simonsen, D. W. Cameron, M. Bosire, and P. Waiyaki. 1988. "Prevention of Transmission of Human Immunodeficiency Virus in Africa." *The Lancet* 2 (8616): 887–890.

Ngugi, E. N., D. Wilson, J. Sebstad, F. A. Plummer, and S. Moses. 1996. "Focused Peer-Mediated Educational Programs among Female Sex Workers." *Journal of Infectious Diseases* 174 (Suppl. 2): S240–247.

NIAID (National Institute of Allergy and Infectious Diseases) and NIH (National Institutes of Health). 2002. "U.S. Health Institutes Release HIV/AIDS Drug Trials Statement." Review of HIVNET 012. Released March 22. Available online at <http://www.usembassy.it/file2002_03/alia/a2032410.htm>. Accessed October 2, 2002.

Nicholas, H. G. 1975. *The United Nations as a Political Institution*. 5th ed. Oxford: Oxford University Press.

Nkya, W. M., S. H. Gillespie, W. Howlett, J. Elford, C. Nyamuryekunge, C. Assenga, and B. Nyombi. 1991. "Sexually Transmitted Diseases in Prostitutes in Moshi and Arusha, North Tanzania." *International Journal of STD & AIDS* 2, no. 6: 432–435.

Nsanze, H., M. V. Fast, L. J. D'Costa, P. Tukei, J. Curran, and A. Ronald. 1981. "Genital Ulcers in Kenya: Clinical and Laboratory Study." *British Journal of Venereal Diseases* 57, no. 6: 378–381.

Nzomo, Maria. 1997. "Kenyan Women in Politics and Public Decision Making." In *African Feminism: The Politics of Survival in Sub-Saharan Africa*, edited by Gwendolyn Mikell. Philadelphia: University of Pennsylvania Press.

Obbo, Christine. 1980. *African Women: Their Struggle for Economic Independence.* London: Zed.

———. 1993. "HIV Transmission through Social and Geographical Networks in Uganda." *Social Science and Medicine* 36, no. 7: 949–955.

Obudho, R. A., and G. O. Aduwo. 1992. "The Nature of the Urbanization Process and Urbanism in the City of Nairobi, Kenya." *African Urban Quarterly* 7, no. 1/2: 50–62.

Odongo, F., and S. B. Ojwang. 1990. "Some Aspects of Teenage Pregnancy in Nairobi: A Prospective Study on Teenage Mothers at Kenyatta National Hospital and Pumwani Maternity Hospital." *East African Medical Journal* 67, no. 6: 432–436.

Ogot, B. A., and W. R. Ochieng, eds. 1995. *Decolonization and Independence in Kenya, 1940–93.* London: James Currey.

Okoko, Tervil. 2002. "Kenya's Raging Debate on Abortion Continues." PANA Daily Newswire, May 15. Available online from the NexisLexis database.

Ong, Aihwa. 1987. *Spirits of Resistance and Capitalist Discipline: Factory Women in Malaysia.* Albany: SUNY Press.

———. 1999. *Flexible Citizenship: The Cultural Logics of Transnationalism.* Durham, N.C.: Duke University Press.

Orvis, Stephen. 2001. "Moral Ethnicity and Political Tribalism in Kenya's 'Virtual Democracy.'" *African Issues* 29, no. 1 and 2: 8–13.

Outwater, Anne. 1996. "The Socioeconomic Impact of AIDS on Women in Tanzania." In *Women's Experiences with HIV/AIDS: An International Perspective,* edited by Lynellen D. Long and E. Maxine Ankrah. New York: Columbia University Press.

Packard, Randall M. 1989. "Epidemiologists, Social Scientists, and the Structure of Medical Research on AIDS in Africa." *Working Papers in African Studies,* no. 137. Boston: Boston University African Studies Center.

Packard, Randall M., and Paul Epstein. 1992. "Medical Research on AIDS in Africa: A Historical Perspective." In *AIDS: The Making of a Chronic Disease,* edited by Elizabeth Fee and Daniel M. Fox. Berkeley: University of California Press.

Palca, Joseph. 1991. "WHO AIDS Program: Moving on a New Track." *Science* 254 (October 25): 511–512.

Panos. 1989. *AIDS in the Third World.* Budapest: Panos Institute.

———. 1990. *Triple Jeopardy: Women and AIDS.* Budapest: Panos Institute.

Parham, D., and R. Conviser. 2002. "A Brief History of the Ryan White CARE Act in the USA and Its Implications for Other Countries." *AIDS Care* 14 (Suppl. 1): S3–S6.

Patton, Cindy. 1990. *Inventing AIDS.* New York: Routledge.

———. 1992. "From Nation to Family: Containing African AIDS." In *Nationalisms and Sexualities,* edited by Andrew Parker, Mary Russo, Doris Summer, and Patricia Yeager. New York: Routledge.

———. 1994. *Last Served: Gendering the HIV Epidemic.* New York: Taylor and Francis.

——. 2002. *Globalizing AIDS*. Minneapolis: University of Minnesota Press.

Pattullo, A., J. Nasio, and M. Malisa. 1993. "Increased HIV-1 Prevalence in Women with Genital Ulcer Disease Presenting to an STD Clinic in Nairobi, Kenya." *International Conference on AIDS* 9, no. 2: 732. Abstract PO-C20 3091.

Petersen, Alan, and Robin Bunton, eds. 1997. *Foucault: Health and Medicine*. London: Routledge.

Pheterson, Gail. 1990. "The Category 'Prostitute' in Scientific Inquiry." *Journal of Sex Research* 27, no. 3: 397–407.

——, ed. 1989. *A Vindication of the Rights of Whores*. Seattle: Seal.

Piot, P., F. A. Plummer, F. S. Mhalu, J. L. Lamboray, J. Chin, and J. M. Mann. 1988. "AIDS: An International Perspective." *Science* 239, no. 4840: 573–579.

Piot, P., F. A. Plummer, M. A. Rey, E. N. Ngugi, C. Rouzioux, J. O. Ndinya-Achola, G. Veracauteren, L. J. D'Costa, M. Laga, and H. Nsanze. 1987. "Retrospective Seroepidemiology of AIDS Virus Infection in Nairobi Populations." *Journal of Infectious Diseases* 155, no. 6: 1108–1112.

Plourde, P., J. Pepin, E. Agoki, A. R. Ronald, J. Ombette, M. Tyndall, M. Cheang, J. O. Ndinya-Achola, L. J. D'Costa, and F. A. Plummer. 1994. "Human Immunodeficiency Virus Type 1 Seroconversion in Women with Genital Ulcers." *Journal of Infectious Diseases* 170, no. 2: 313–317.

Plourde, P. J., F. A. Plummer, J. Pepin, E. Agoki, G. Moss, J. Ombette, and A. R. Ronald. 1992. "Human Immunodeficiency Virus Type 1 Infection in Women Attending a Sexually Transmitted Diseases Clinic in Kenya." *Journal of Infectious Diseases* 166, no. 1: 86–92.

Plummer, Francis A., Roel A. Coutinho, Elizabeth N. Ngugi, and Stephen Moses. 1998. "Sex Workers and Their Clients in the Epidemiology and Control of Sexually Transmitted Diseases." In *Sexually Transmitted Diseases*, 3d ed., edited by Holmes, Sparling, and Wasserheit.

Plummer, F. A., L. J. D'Costa, H. Nsanze, J. Dylewski, P. Karasira, and A. R. Ronald. 1983. "Epidemiology of Chancroid and *Haemophilus ducreyi* in Nairobi, Kenya." *The Lancet* 2, no. 8362: 1293–1295.

Plummer, F. A., L. J. D'Costa, H. Nsanze, P. Karasira, I. W. MacLean, P. Piot, and A. R. Ronald. 1985. "Clinical and Microbiologic Studies of Genital Ulcers in Kenyan Women." *Sexually Transmitted Diseases* 12, no. 4: 193–197.

Plummer, F. A., N. J. Nagelkerke, S. Moses, J. O. Ndinya-Achola, J. Bwayo, and E. Ngugi. 1991. "The Importance of Core Groups in the Epidemiology and Control of HIV-1 Infection." *AIDS* 5 (Suppl. 1): S169–176.

Plummer, F. A., J. N. Simonsen, D. W. Cameron, J. O. Ndinya-Achola, J. K. Kreiss, M. N. Gakinya, P. Waiyaki, M. Cheang, P. Piot, and A. R. Ronald. 1991. "Cofactors in Male-Female Sexual Transmission of Human Immunodeficiency Virus Type 1." *Journal of Infectious Diseases* 163, no. 2: 233–239.

Poster, Winifred R. 2002. "Racialism, Sexuality, and Masculinity: Gendering 'Global Ethnography' of the Workplace." *Social Politics* 9, no. 1: 126–158.

Pratt, Mary Louise. 1992. *Imperial Eyes: Travel Writing and Transculturation*. New York: Routledge.

Public Citizen. 1998a. "Health Group Files Suit Over NIH Experiments on HIV-

Positive Women in Developing Countries." Press release, March 18. Available online at <http://www.citizen.org/pressroom/print_release.cfm?ID=241>. Accessed March 15, 2003.

———. 1998b. "Health Group Attacks Second Generation of Unethical Perinatal Trials in Africa: Researchers to Deny HIV-Positive Pregnant Women Effective, Less Expensive Drug Regimens." Press release, July 1. Available online at <http://www.citizen.org/pressroom/print_release.cfm?ID=320>. Accessed March 15, 2003.

———. 1999. "Scientists Seek to Justify and Continue Unethical Research by Gutting International Ethical Guidelines." Press Release, August 11. Available online at <http://www.citizen.org/pressroom/print_release.cfm?ID=348>. Accessed March 15, 2003.

Quinn, T. C., J. M. Mann, J. W. Curran, and P. Piot. 1986. "AIDS in Africa: An Epidemiologic Paradigm." *Science* 234, no. 4779: 955–963.

Renaud, Michelle Lewis. 1997. *Women at the Crossroads: A Prostitute Community's Response to AIDS in Urban Senegal.* Amsterdam: Overseas Publishers Association/Gordon and Breach Publishers.

Robertson, Claire. 1997. *Trouble Showed the Way: Women, Men, and Trade in the Nairobi Area, 1890–1990.* Bloomington: Indiana University Press.

Rodriguez, Bob. 1997. "Biomedical Models of HIV and Women." In *The Gender Politics of HIV/AIDS in Women: Perspectives on the Pandemic in the United States,* edited by Nancy Goldstein and Jennifer L. Marlowe. New York: New York University Press.

Rodriguez-Trias, Helen, and Carola Marte. 1994. "The Role of Nurses in the HIV Epidemic." In *Women Resisting AIDS,* edited by Schneider and Stoller.

Ronald, Alan, and William Albritton. 1992. "Chancroid and *Haemophilus ducreyi.*" In *Sexually Transmitted Diseases,* 2d ed., edited by Holmes.

———. 1998. "Chancroid and *Haemophilus ducreyi.*" In *Sexually Transmitted Diseases,* 3d ed., edited by Holmes, Sparling, and Wasserheit.

Ronald, A., F. Plummer, E. Ngugi, E. O. Ndinya-Achola, P. Piot, J. Kreiss, and R. Brunham. 1991. "The Nairobi STD Program: An International Partnership." *Infectious Disease Clinics of North America* 5, no. 2: 337–352.

Sabatier, Renée. 1988. *Blaming Others: Prejudice, Race, and Worldwide AIDS.* Budapest: Panos Institute.

Said, Edward W. 1978. *Orientalism.* New York: Pantheon Books.

Sandbrook, Richard. 1985. *The Politics of Africa's Economic Stagnation.* Cambridge: Cambridge University Press.

Sanders, David, and Abdulrahman Sambo. 1991. "AIDS in Africa: The Implications of Economic Recession and Structural Adjustment." *Health Policy and Planning* 6, no. 2: 157–165.

Sassen, Saskia. 1998. *Globalization and Its Discontents.* New York: The New Press.

Schatzburg, Michael. 1987. *The Political Economy of Kenya.* New York: Praeger.

Scheper-Hughes, Nancy. 1992. *Death without Weeping: The Violence of Everyday Life in Brazil.* Berkeley: University of California Press.

Schick, Suzaynn. 1997. "Ethics in the Age of AIDS." *Synapse,* October 30. Available online at <http://www.ucsf.edu/synapse/archives/oct30.97/schick.html>. Accessed March 23, 2002.

Schiebinger, Londa L. 1993. *Nature's Body: Gender in the Making of Modern Science.* Boston: Beacon.

Schneider, Beth E., and Nancy E. Stoller, eds. 1994. *Women Resisting AIDS: Feminist Strategies of Empowerment.* Philadelphia: Temple University Press.

Schoepf, Brooke Grundfest. 1988. "Women, AIDS, and Economic Crisis in Central Africa." *Canadian Journal of African Studies* 22, no. 3: 625–644.

———. 1997. "AIDS, Gender, and Sexuality during Africa's Economic Crisis." In *African Feminism: The Politics of Survival in Sub-Saharan Africa,* edited by Gwendolyn Mikell. Philadelphia: University of Pennsylvania Press.

Setel, Philip W. 1999. *A Plague of Paradoxes: AIDS, Culture, and Demography in Northern Tanzania.* Chicago: University of Chicago Press.

Shaw, Carolyn Martin. 1995. *Colonial Inscriptions: Race, Sex, and Class in Kenya.* Minneapolis: University of Minnesota Press.

Shelton, Deborah. 1998. "CDC, NIH Halt Controversial Use of Placebos in AZT Trials." *American Medical News* 41, no. 11. Available online at <http://www.ama-assn.org/special/hiv/newsline/special/amnews/placebo.htm>. Accessed March 23, 2002.

Simonsen, J. N., D. W. Cameron, M. N. Gakinya, J. O. Ndinya-Achola, L. J. D'Costa, P. Karasira, M. Cheang, A. R. Ronald, P. Piot, and F. A. Plummer. 1988. "Human Immunodeficiency Virus Infection among Men with Sexually Transmitted Diseases: Experience from a Center in Africa." *New England Journal of Medicine* 319, no. 5: 274–278.

Simonsen, J. N., et al. 1990. "HIV Infection among Lower Socioeconomic Strata Prostitutes in Nairobi." *AIDS* 4, no. 2: 139–144.

Siringi, Samuel. 2001a. "Generic Drugs Battle Moves from South Africa to Kenya." *The Lancet* 357 (May 19): 1600.

———. 2001b. "Kenya Forms Taskforce to Tackle AIDS." *The Lancet* 358 (July 14): 133.

Smith, Susan L. 1995. *Sick and Tired of Being Sick and Tired: Black Women's Health Activism in America, 1890–1950.* Philadelphia: University of Pennsylvania Press.

Somerville, Siobhan. 1997. "Scientific Racism and the Invention of the Homosexual Body." In *The Gender/Sexuality Reader,* edited by Roger N. Lancaster and Micaela di Leonardo. New York: Routledge.

Sontag, Susan. 1989. *AIDS and Its Metaphors.* New York: Farrar, Strauss, and Giroux.

Spivak, Gayatri. 1988. "Can the Subaltern Speak?" In *Marxism and the Interpretation of Culture,* edited by Cary Nelson and Lawrence Grossberg. Urbana: University of Illinois Press.

Stepan, Nancy Leys. 1982. *The Idea of Race in Science: Great Britain, 1800–1960.* Hamdon, Conn.: Archon Books.

———. 1996. "Race and Gender: The Role of Analogy in Science." In *Feminism and Science,* edited by Nancy Tuana. Bloomington: Indiana University Press.

Stepan, Nancy Leys, and Sander Gilman. 1991. "Appropriating the Idioms of Science: The Rejection of Scientific Racism." In *The Bounds of Race: Perspectives on Hegemony and Resistance,* edited by Dominick LaCapra. Ithaca, N.Y.: Cornell University Press.

Stichter, Sharon. 1985. *Migrant Laborers.* Cambridge: Press Syndicate of the University of Cambridge.

Stoler, Ann Laura. 1989a. "Making Empire Respectable: The Politics of Race and Sexual Morality in 20th Century Colonial Cultures." *American Ethnologist* 16, no. 4: 634–660.

———. 1989b. "Rethinking Colonial Categories: European Communities and the Boundaries of Rule." *Comparative Studies in Society and History* 31, no. 1 (January): 134–161.

———. 1991. "Carnal Knowledge and Imperial Power: Gender, Race, and Morality in Colonial Asia." In *Gender at the Crossroads of Knowledge,* edited by Micaela di Leonardo. Berkeley: University of California Press.

———. 1995. *Race and the Education of Desire: Foucault's History of Sexuality and the Colonial Order of Things.* Durham, N.C.: Duke University Press.

Swarns, Rachel L. 2001. "AIDS Drug Battle Deepens in Africa." *New York Times,* March 8, A1.

Tabet, Paola. 1989. "'I'm the meat, I'm the knife': Sexual Service, Migration and Repression in Some African Societies." In *A Vindication of the Rights of Whores,* edited by Pheterson.

Tandia, Oumar. 1998. "Prostitution in Senegal." In *Global Sex Workers: Rights, Resistance, and Redefinition,* edited by Kemala Kempadoo and Jo Doezema. New York: Routledge.

Temmerman, M., F. A. Plummer, N. B. Mirza, J. O. Ndinya-Achola, I. A. Wamola, N. Nagelkerke, R. C. Brunham, and P. Piot. 1990. "Infection with HIV as a Risk Factor for Adverse Obstetrical Outcome." *AIDS* 4, no. 11: 1087–1093.

Temmerman, M., and R. W. Ryder. 1991. "The Effect of HIV-1 Infection during Pregnancy and the Perinatal Period on Maternal and Child Health in Africa." *AIDS* 5 (Suppl. 1): S75–85.

Thomas-Slayter, Barbara. 1991. "Class, Community and the Kenyan State: Community Mobilization in the Context of Global Politics." *International Journal of Politics, Culture, and Society* 4, no. 3: 301–321.

Throup, David. 1993. "Elections and Political Legitimacy in Kenya." *Africa* 63, no. 3: 371–396.

Treichler, Paula A. 1988a. "AIDS, Gender, and Biomedical Discourse: Current Contests for Meaning." In *AIDS: The Burdens of History,* edited by Elizabeth Fee and Daniel M. Fox. Berkeley: University of California Press.

———. 1988b. "AIDS, Homophobia, and Biomedical Discourse: An Epidemic of Signification." *Cultural Studies* 1, no. 3: 263–305.

———. 1999. *How to Have Theory in an Epidemic: Cultural Chronicles of AIDS.* Durham, N.C.: Duke University Press.

Turshen, Meredith. 1999. *Privatizing Health Services in Africa.* New Brunswick, N.J.: Rutgers University Press.

Ulin, Priscilla R. 1992. "African Women and AIDS: Negotiating Behavioral Change." *Social Science and Medicine* 34, no. 1: 63–73.

UNAIDS (Joint United Nations Programme on HIV/AIDS). 1999. "Questions and Answers: Mother-to-Child Transmission (MTCT) of HIV." August 5. Available online at <http://www.unaids.org/publications/documents/mtct/qaweb99.html>. Accessed March 15, 2003.

UNAIDS and WHO. 2002. *AIDS Epidemic Update: December, 2002.* Geneva: UNAIDS.

U.S. Census Bureau. 2002. *HIV/AIDS Surveillance Data Base: June, 2002.* Available on CD-ROM.

U.S. Public Health Service, National Pediatric and Family HIV Resource Center. 1999. "Women with HIV: A U.S. Fact Sheet." Available online at <http://www.pedhivaids.org/fact/women_fact_us.html>. Accessed October 21, 2002.

Van der Horst, Charles. 2002. "African Diary." *Independent Weekly* (Durham, North Carolina), June 19–25, 1.

Vaughan, Megan. 1991. *Curing Their Ills.* Cambridge: Polity.

Verhagen, A. R., and W. Gemert. 1972. "Social and Epidemiological Determinants of Gonorrhoea in an East African Country." *British Journal of Venereal Disease* 48, no. 4: 277–286.

Verhagen, A. R., M. Van der Ham, A. L. Heimans, O. Kranendonk, and A. N. Maina. 1971. "Diminished Antibiotic Sensitivity of *Neisseria gonorrhoeae* in Urban and Rural Areas in Kenya." *Bulletin of the World Health Organization* 45: 707–717.

Vick, Karl. 2001. "AIDS Vaccine Hopes Rise from Africa: 'Killer T-Cells' Seem to Naturally Protect Some Prostitutes." *The Washington Post*, May 11, A1.

Wakhweya, Angela M. 1995. "Structural Adjustment and Health." *British Medical Journal* 311: 71–72.

Walkowitz, Judith. 1980. *Prostitution and Victorian Society: Women, Class, and the State.* Cambridge: Cambridge University Press.

Wallman, Sandra. 1996. *Kampala Women Getting By: Wellbeing in the Time of AIDS.* London: James Currey.

Watney, Simon. 1989a. "AIDS, Language and the Third World." In *Taking Liberties: AIDS and Cultural Politics*, edited by Erika Carter and Simon Watney. London: Serpent's Tail.

———. 1989b. "Missionary Positions: AIDS, 'Africa,' and Race." *Differences* 1, no. 1: 83–100.

Watts, D. Heather, and Robert C. Brunham. 1998. "Sexually Transmitted Diseases including HIV in Pregnancy." In *Sexually Transmitted Diseases*, 3d ed., edited by Holmes, Sparling, and Wasserheit.

White, Luise. 1990. *The Comforts of Home: Prostitution in Colonial Nairobi.* Chicago: University of Chicago Press.

WHO (World Health Organization). 1978. *Primary Health Care.* Geneva: World Health Organization.

———. 1984. "Acquired Immune Deficiency Syndrome: An Assessment of the Present Situation in the World." *Bulletin of the World Health Organization* 62, no. 3: 419–432.

——. 1986. "Acquired Immune Deficiency Syndrome (AIDS)." *Weekly Epidemiological Record* 61, no. 5: 35.

——. 1987. *Global AIDS Strategy*. Geneva: World Health Organization.

——. 1988. *Guidelines for the Development of a National AIDS Prevention and Control Programme*. Geneva: World Health Organization.

——. 1990a. "AIDS and the Status of Women: Challenges and Perspectives for the 1990s." *WHO Features* 149 (October).

——. 1990b. "Women and AIDS in the 1990s: New WHO Analysis Sees Rapid Worsening of AIDS Impact." *WHO Features* 151 (November).

——. 1992a. *Global Strategy for the Prevention and Control of AIDS: 1992 Update*. Geneva: World Health Organization.

——. 1992b. "New AIDS Strategy Aimed More at Women." *World Health Forum* 13: 91.

——. 1993a. "WHO Sponsored Study Finds No Evidence for Kemron Claims." Press release, June 7.

WHO (World Health Organization) and UNAIDS (Joint UN Programme on HIV/AIDS). 2002. "WHO and UNAIDS Continue to Support Use of Nevirapine for Prevention of Mother-to-Child HIV Transmission." Joint WHO/UNAIDS press statement, March 22. Available online at <http://www.who.int/inf/en/WHO-UNAIDstate2002.html>. Accessed March 27, 2002.

Willerford, Dennis M., Job J. Bwayo, Michelle Hensel, Wilfred Emonyi, Francis A. Plummer, Elizabeth N. Ngugi, Nico Nagelkerke, W. Michael Gallatin, and Joan Kreiss. 1993. "Human Immunodeficiency Virus Infection among High-Risk Seronegative Prostitutes in Nairobi." *Journal of Infectious Diseases* 167 (June): 1414–1417.

Wilson, David, Paul Cawthorne, Nathan Ford, and Saree Aongsonwang. 1999. "Global Trade and Access to Medicines: AIDS Treatments in Thailand." *The Lancet* 354 (November 27): 9193.

Wolpe, Harold. 1972. "Capitalism and Cheap Labour-Power in South Africa: From Segregation to Apartheid." *Economy and Society* 1: 425–456.

Wrong, Michela. 1995. "Kenya Tests Limits of Foreign Goodwill." *Financial Times* (London), May 30, 6.

Yuval-Davis, Nora, and Floya Anthias, eds. 1989. *Woman-Nation-State*. London: Macmillan.

de Zalduondo, Barbara O. 1991. "Prostitution Viewed Cross-Culturally." *The Journal of Sex Research* 28, no. 2: 223–248.

Zierler, Sally. 1994. "Women, Sex and HIV." *Epidemiology* 5: 565–567.

Unpublished Documents

CIDA (Canadian International Development Agency). 1990. "Strengthening STD Control in Kenya." CIDA Project Number 524/16173. Unpublished report.

——. 1992. "Strengthening STD/AIDS Control in Kenya." CIDA Project Number 524/16173. Unpublished report.

————. n.d. Flowchart for treatment of common sexually transmitted diseases. In author's possession.

Government of Kenya and WHO. 1987. "The Kenya National Programme Plan on AIDS, 1987–1991." Geneva: WHO.

————. 1989. "The Kenya National AIDS Control Programme Review, March 27 to April 4."

————. 1992. "The Second Five Year Medium Term Plan for AIDS Control, 1992–1996." Geneva: WHO.

Merson, Michael H. 1991. Keynote speech to the VI International Conference on AIDS in Africa. Dakar, Senegal, December 16.

UNAIDS (United Nations Programme on HIV/AIDS). 2000. "Ethical Considerations in HIV Preventive Vaccine Research." UNAIDS guidance document. Geneva: UNAIDS.

UNECOSOC (United Nations Economic and Social Council). 1994. "Joint and Co-sponsored United Nations Programme on Human Immunodeficiency Virus/Acquired Immunodeficiency Syndrome (HIV/AIDS)." Resolution E94RO24. July 26.

USAID (United States Agency for International Development). 1991. "An Assessment of the Economic Impact of AIDS in Kenya." Report prepared by AIDSTECH and Family Health International. Mimeo.

WHO (World Health Organization). 1989. Global Programme on AIDS and Sexually Transmitted Diseases Programme. "Consensus Statement from the Consultation on HIV Epidemiology and Prostitution." Geneva, July 3–6. WHO/GPA/INF/89.11.

————. 1990c. "Global Strategy for the Prevention and Control of AIDS: Paris Declaration on Women, Children and the Acquired Immune Deficiency Syndrome (AIDS)." Eighty-fifth Session of the Executive Board, Provisional Agenda Item 16. January 17. EB85/INF.DOC/3.

————. 1990d. "Global Strategy for the Prevention and Control of AIDS: Report of the Director-General to the Eighty-seventh Session of the Executive Board." Geneva, December 12. Geneva: WHO.

————. 1993b. "Draft Global Strategic Plan: Women and AIDS." Prepared by the Women's Internal Working Group, Kathleen Cravero, and Priscilla Alexander. Geneva, May 25. In author's possession.

Index

abortion, 15, 170n24

Achmat, Zakie, 136

"African AIDS" paradigm, 47–50, 70, 84, 89, 91, 99, 165n21. *See also* scientific metaphors

"African" defined, 148n8, 151n1

African Regional Office (WHO), 55

AIDS activists, 10, 12, 49, 107. *See also* AIDS Coalition to Unleash Power (ACT UP); Treatment Action Campaign (TAC)

AIDS Clinical Trial Group 076, 129–130, 132–133

AIDS Coalition to Unleash Power (ACT UP), 143–144

AIDS treatment drugs: AZT, *see* azidothymidine (AZT); chlorhexidine, 134; Kemron, 73; nevirapine, 135–136, 140, 172–173n11, 173n13; protease inhibitors, 135, 139

Alexander, Priscilla, ix–x, 161n32

American Foundation for AIDS Research, 81

antibiotics, 33, 37, 41, 110, 162n5

anti-imperialist critiques of science, 82–83

anti-racist critiques of science, 162n4

azidothymidine (AZT): and absence of studies of effects on pregnant and lactating women, 139–140; African states' inability to afford, 136, 141; clinical

trials of, 13, 127–132, 134, 136, 140; debate about who should fund, 135; ineffectiveness of, 171n2; international health officials' reliance on, 135, 139; TAC's efforts to obtain in South Africa, 173n13; use of in United States, 171n2, 173n14

Bamako Initiative, 115, 169n8

Belgium, 36–37, 82, 97, 134, 158n6, 161n22

Bestlands Estate, 108, 112

Bestlands Health Centre: clientele of, 109; described, 108; maternalism at, 121; nurses help women conceal contraceptives from sexual partners, 148n11; nurses' analysis of male heterosexuality, 117; and reliance on Canadian-led research team for funding, 6, 113; and responsibility to provide primary health care services, 1, 13, 112–113; and selective decisions about services, 5, 122; shortage of supplies at, 109–111; and treatment by Kenyan state, 115; and view of female clients as powerless, 2, 4

binary thinking, 164–165n18; and drug use, 165n18; and male sexuality, 41; and race, 165n18; and sexual orientation, 165n18. *See also* whore/mother dichotomy

Index

Index

"high-frequency transmitter" model, 86–91, 93–94, 97, 100–102, 104; "patterns" of AIDS transmission, 51–52, 163n10; recruitment and activation, 101; reservoir, 88, 90, 94, 100, 163n9; virus shedding, 91, 101

Searching for Hawa's Secret (documentary), 105–106

Setel, Philip, 90

sex workers: complexity of, 96; critique the WHO, 53–54; discriminated against by medical community, 58; and founding of Nairobi, 103, 166–167n29; harassment at public clinics, 44; and "high-frequency transmitter" model, 88; Kenyan state's harassment of, 15; Kenyan state's regulation of, 154n16; as objects of biomedical research, 34, 78, 90, 105–106; and problems with biomedical models about, 99; rates of HIV infection in Nairobi, 63; in Senegal, 164n17; in South Africa, 167n30; WHO defines as separate from mothers, 56; WHO feminists lobby on behalf of, 72. *See also* prostitutes

Sexually Transmitted Diseases, 86

smallpox, 55, 160n11

South Africa: and AZT trials, 129, 132–133; battles multinational pharmaceutical companies, 20, 141, 143; and denial of AIDS, 18, 135–136; rates of HIV infection among pregnant women, 131; Treatment Action Campaign challenges, 137. *See also* Mbeki, President Thabo; Treatment Action Campaign (TAC)

Special Program on AIDS (SPA), 54–55

squatter settlements, 29, 102, 108

structural adjustment programs, 8, 16, 32, 58, 60, 62, 142

Swiss Red Cross, 37

Switzerland, 47

syphilis: and Canadian-led research team's resources for treating, 82; and co-factor theory of HIV transmission, 94, 154n20; in colonial Kenya, 20, 25, 88; and drug shortages in clinics, 35, 40; and misdiagnosis as chancroid, 155n25; and racist medical models, 28, 30; resistance to penicillin, 154n14; and stigmatizing medical models, 100;

testing for, 32, 114; treatment of at Bestlands Health Centre, 168n6

Tanzania, 18, 54, 90, 93, 129, 131–132, 139

technical assistance and national policy, 59

tourism: and concerns over contaminated blood, 64–65; and denial of AIDS in Kenya, 17, 52, 63; and globalism, 8, 11; mentioned, 22, 85; and WHO's entry into Kenya, 63, 161n19

training of clinic staff about HIV/AIDS: Canadian-led research team and, 79–80, 82, 113–114, 155n31; dependence of Kenyans on donors for, 5, 31, 36–37, 64, 73, 169n10; funded by Kenyan state, 17; of nurses in Nairobi's clinics, 7, 33, 168n6; and shortage of medical supplies in Nairobi's clinics, 111; and shortage of staff in Nairobi's clinics, 109–110

Treatment Action Campaign (TAC), 136–137, 142–143, 173n13

tribal affiliation. *See* ethnic groups in Kenya

tuberculosis, 8, 23, 26, 100

Tuskegee Syphilis Study, 131

Uganda, 18, 54, 88–89, 129, 132–133, 139, 141, 158n3, 161n19

United Kingdom. *See* Britain

United Nations, 73, 112, 172n7

United Nations Development Programme (UNDP), 62, 73

United States Agency for International Development (USAID), 16–17, 37, 58, 138, 150n18

University of Antwerp, 80

University of London, 36

University of Manitoba, 33, 80–81, 115, 116

University of Nairobi, 35, 78, 81, 92, 110, 113, 156n31

University of Washington (Seattle), 80–81

U.S. Food and Drug Administration, 171n2

U.S. National Institutes of Health, 81

violence against women. *See* domestic abuse

"virus shedding" metaphor, 91, 101. *See also* scientific metaphors

whore/mother dichotomy, 57–58, 97–99

Wilfert, Dr. Catherine, 131

Karen M. Booth is Associate Professor of Women's Studies at the University of North Carolina at Chapel Hill.